William Augustus Evans

Notes on Pathology

For Students Use

William Augustus Evans

Notes on Pathology
For Students Use

ISBN/EAN: 9783742830050

Manufactured in Europe, USA, Canada, Australia, Japa

Cover: Foto ©Lupo / pixelio.de

Manufactured and distributed by brebook publishing software
(www.brebook.com)

William Augustus Evans

Notes on Pathology

NOTES ON PATHOLOGY

--

FOR STUDENTS' USE.

BY

W. A. EVANS, B. SC., M. D.

PROFESSOR OF PATHOLOGY MEDICAL SCHOOL OF THE UNIVERSITY
OF ILLINOIS: PROFESSOR OF PATHOLOGY MILWAUKEE
MEDICAL COLLEGE; PATHOLOGIST COLUMBUS
MEDICAL LABORATORY, ETC.

CHICAGO:
CHICAGO MEDICAL BOOK CO.,
35-37 Randolph Street,
1898.

PREFACE

This has been written by a teacher for students. It does not pretend to originality. Green, Hamilton, Zeigler, Orth, Woodhead, Cabot have been freely consulted. My thanks are due Drs. L. J. Mitchell and C. C. O'Byrne.

W. A. EVANS.

TABLE OF CONTENTS.

NOTES ON PATHOLOGY.

Pathology is the science of the lesions found in tissues, both as a cause of, and as a result of disease.

Pathological anatomy is the science of the lesions recognizable by the unaided eye.

Pathological histology is the science of the lesions recognizable by the microscope.

Pathological processes divide themselves into:

1. Inflammations.
2. Degenerations.
3. Tumor growths.

INFLAMMATIONS.

Inflammations are pathological exaggerations of the normal processes of repair. Every inflammation depends upon irritation. In every irritation there are two factors: (1) the irritant, and (2) the cell irritated.

The Cell Irritated. As a rule, the more highy differentiated a cell, the greater its irritability.

All cells spring originally from the ovum: they arrange themselves into three layers, and these further develop into tissues and organs. The fact that the cells of a certain organ do a certain work is proof that the demand for that work is an irritant to those cells; e. g., the fact that the kidney epithelium secretes urine is proof that these epithelial cells are irritated by the antecedents of urine. Urea is, then, a special irritant to kidney epithelium, and only a general irritant to the other tissues of the body.

The parenchyma is the working part of an organ. It is immaterial from what blastic layer it is derived; it is the most easily irritated of the tissues of that organ.

Irritants are general and special: A general irritant is one that is irritating in proportion to the irritability of the cells. Special irritants are those that only irritate certain cells; e. g., the irritant causing destruction of liver epithelium in acute yellow atrophy.

Inflammations are divisible into two great classes:

1. Productive.
2. Destructive.

Physiological irritation is responsible for function. Moderate pathological irritation

gives productive inflammation; this, carried one step further, gives destructive inflammation.

Productive inflammations are divisible into:

1. Non-exudative.
2. Exudative.

The elements that make up a tissue can, then, be divided for our purposes into:

1. The local cells.
2. The vessels.

If an irritant affect the first only, we have a non-uxudative productive inflammation. If it affect the first and second, we have an exudative productive inflammation. If it involve the second only, we have an angio-neurotic œdema (urticaria), a condition scarcely consequential enough to be considered in this connection.

When cells are irritated beyond the usual limits, and yet short of destruction, partial or complete, they divide by:

1. Direct division, in which the nucleus and the cell protoplasm divide simultaneously; this is unusual. Or by:

2. Indirect division, called also mitosis and karyokinesis. In this the nucleus first divides, then the cell protoplasm. The nucleus is made up of a threadwork and a delicate semi-

fluid interfibrillar substance. This skeinwork first arranges itself regularly, then unravels, and the two stars assume opposite poles of the nucleus; then the spongioplasm divides, then the cell protoplasm cleaves. The new skein in the new nucleus assumes then its irregular resting stage. This is the usual method of dividing.

TRANSUDATIONS.

A transudation is constantly taking place from the vessels. So long as the capillaries and lymphatics bear off the transudate as fast as it pours out, no accumulation takes place. This is physiological transudation, and is the means of much of nutrition.

Pathological transudates are divisible into (1) active and (2) passive.

Passive transudation is due to mechanical disturbance of the relation between heart force and the opposing forces. Examples: œdema, ascites.

Active transudations, called exudations, are due to exaggerated permeability of the capillary wall as a result of inflammation. A vasomotor nerve irritated causes the circular muscular fiber of the vessel to contract, the lumen is lessened, the current rapidity is increased If the irritation is increased or continued, the nerve is paralyzed, the fiber relaxes, the

lumen is increased; the normal blood current arrangement (from center out—red cells, red cells and whites, plasma, wall) is lost; leucocytes gather along the wall; the irritated endothelial cells contract and become cubical, and stomata opened at the points of juncture with other cells; through these openings the exudate passes. In ordinary transudation the larger part of the plasma passes through the endothelial cells and is changed thereby; the process is akin to a secretion or a selective action.—Plasma goes through with greatest readiness, therefore, in mild vasomotor irritation the exudate consists of plasma only; more violent irritation gives plasma and leucocytes, and if still more violent gives plasma, leucocytes and red cells.

NON-EXUDATIVE PRODUCTIVE INFLAMMATION.

This variety of inflammation is of no great significance unless there is an appreciable accumulation of tissue elements; therefore, it demands a mild irritation, long continued. It can involve highly differentiated cells alone, in which event the more lowly differentiated connective tissue is unaffected. Generally it involves the more lowly differentiated connective tissue. In this event the more highly dif-

ferentiated forces are sometimes unaffected. sometimes proliferating, and sometimes undergoing some of the varieties of destructive inflammation, dependent upon whether the irritant is very irritating to them or not. Usually the state is that of cloudy swelling. The irritant must be mild, else it will involve the vaso-motor apparatus. It must be long continued in order that production may be appreciable. The irritant, again, must be mild in order to be long continued, for more violent irritation set in motion processes that limit or annul them.

For this reason, non-exudative productive inflammations are usually due to alcohols, leucomaines, and the milder toxalbumins. There is a marked production of new connective tissue; this starts as young round cells, which develop into spindles, and then into fibrillated fibers. Bear in mind the tendency of this new pathological connective tissue to contract and pucker. This contraction is responsible for pressure atrophy in the included tissues. This process is not an even one; it is usually in bands or wedges, dependent on vessel arrangement.

The lessons to learn are:

1. Pathological connective tissue contracts as it matures.

2. That while the lowly differentiated cells are dividing—actively increasing—the same irritation may cause the highly differentiated cells to proliferate or to break down.

EXUDATIVE PRODUCTIVE INFLAMMATIONS.

The irritant affects the vaso-motor apparatus and the local cells. The highly differentiated may be proliferating, but are usually undergoing some form of destructive inflammation, such as cloudy swelling. The lowly differentiated cells proliferate very actively, especially in the vicinity of the poison. The vessels are exuding plasma, leucocytes and red cells, all or either. This exudate overshadows the new cells born of the local cells.

These inflammations are generally more violent and always shorter lived. In this variety are found the classical symptoms of inflammation:

Pain, from pressure on nerve endings;

Heat, from increased metabolism;

Redness, from the presence of blood;

Swelling, from the accumulation of exudate and blood in the part;

Impairment of function, by reason (1) swelling, and (2) inflammatory changes in the functioning elements.

These inflammations lend themselves easily to supperative processes. The irritant subsiding, the vessel tone returns; the unimpaired leucocytes get back into the circulation; the new cells and the impaired leucocytes undergo granular degeneration and absorption by leucocytes.

DESTRUCTIVE INFLAMMATIONS.

1.   Cloudy Swelling—a form of inflammatory degeneration in which granules precipitate in the substance of the semi-liquid protoplasm.

2.   Fatty Degeneration—an inflammatory degeneration following the first mentioned, in which portions of the albuminous protoplasm is converted into fat.

3.   Granular Degeneration—necrosis — a breaking down of the albuminous cells, a loss of organic form. The nucleus persists for a while, but it, too, breaks down. In some areas such a pultaceous mass is called atheroma.

4.   Caseation—the liquids absorb and leave the granules behind.

5.   Liquefaction—due to digestion of the dead masses.

6.   Calcification.—In the process of break-

ing down. organic acids result. These combine with the calcium of the plasma and tissue juices to form calcium salts. Calcification is secondary to necrosis.

7. Suppuration.—Death and partial digestion by the poison of. not only the fixed cells and their offspring, but of wandering cells attracted to the focus of poison—chemotaxis. Chemical irritants disassociated from bacteria can produce suppuration; but practically the only suppurations are those of bacterial origin. In killing and digesting the leucocyte and inflammatory connective tissue cell, much of the poison is destroyed, and new poison requires the presence of secreting organisms.— If these phagocytes destroy the cocci, the process terminates. If the local tissues become habituated to the poison, the process ends. If the cocci become attenuated from soaking in their own poisons, the process ends.

Suppuration on a surface is called an ulcer; below a surface it is called an abscess.

RESOLUTION.

The irritation having subsided, the amount of dead and functionally inactive tissue is so small that the phagocytes can assimilate or transport it.

DEGENERATIONS AND INFILTRATIONS.

A degeneration is the substitution for a higher protoplasm of a substance lower in the chemical scale. It is, therefore, a molecular transformation, and does not apply to the substitution of one class of cells by another.

An infiltration is the addition to a higher protoplasm of a substance lower in the scale without any change in the higher protoplasm.

The line between these processes is difficult to draw.

The degenerations are:

1. Cloudy swelling.
2. Fatty degeneration.
3. Necrosis.
4. Coagulation necrosis.
5. Caseation.
6. Gangrene.

The infiltrations are:

1. Fatty.
2. Glycogenic.
3. Serous.

The mixed degenerations and infiltrations are those in which there is some preliminary change in the cell protoplasm, but in which the amount of infiltered substance overshadows the primary change. These are:

1. Amyloid.
2. Mucoid.
3. Colloid.
4. Hyaline.

Degenerations are due to faults of nutrition as to (a) quantity, and (b) quality. A degeneration may accompany inflammation, in which event the quality of the pabulum is at fault, as in cloudy swelling due to irritant poisons. The degenerations that may be inflammatory are cloudy swelling, fatty degeneration and all forms of necrosis.

Or, it may not be connected with inflammation, in which event the quantity of nutrition is less than the cell requires for its purpose.

The degenerations that may be non-inflammatory are fatty, amyloid, mucoid, colloid, serous.

The inflammatory infiltrations are serous.

The non-inflammatory infiltrations are fatty, glycogenous and serous.

It is to be borne in mind that certain of the

degenerations and infiltrations are under certain circumstances entirely physiological For example, milk is a composite of a watery exudate and the epithelial cells of the mammary gland in a state of fatty degeneration. , The sebaceous secretion of the skin is of the same nature.

ALBUMINOUS DEGENERATION.

Synonym: Cloudy swelling.

Causes: Nutrition minus—deficiency in quality; nutritive fluids contain a poison.

Nature: An inflammatory degeneration.

Results histologically: Return to normal, fatty degeneration, or, if process is more violent, necrosis.

Effects physiologically: Loss of function.

Gross appearance: Organ is swollen, paler than normal.

Microscopic appearance: Nucleus is obscured in varying degree; may not be apparent, may be incapable of taking stain, may have disappeared; cell usually swollen, granular; granules small, not highly refractile. Chemically, cell stains poorly, granules soluble in acetic acid. Method: Place a few teased cells on a slide in physiological salt solution; cover; run under cover a drop of 1

per cent. solution of acetic acid; granules disappear.

Nature of process: The increase in size is due to absorption of water. The granules consist of albuminous or albuminoid material, lower in the chemical scale than the normal protoplasm.

FATTY DEGENERATION.

Synonyms: None.

Causes: Nutrition minus, either lack of food supply or toxæmia.

Origin: May be inflammatory, in which event it is preceded by albuminous degeneration, or it may be non-inflammatory.

Results histologically: Return to normal; necrosis and the resulting possibilities of an area of necrosis.

Effects: Loss of function, partial or complete.

Anatomy: Organ pale, not much altered in size.

Microscopic appearance: (Comparison with albuminous degeneration.) Nucleus much less obscured; granules larger, may be globules; granules refract light more.

Chemically: Teased elements show granules or globules of fat; replace salt solution

by ether; the granules are dissolved; stain with a one-fifth of 1 per cent. solution of osmic acid, granules become black. Into teased specimen run 1 per cent. acetic acid, no change is observed; specimens fixed, hardened, embedded, stained and mounted show clear vesicles where the fat originally was.

Nature of process: This represents a retrograde process wherein the higher protoplasm is replaced by fat: This fat is at first in small granules and these coalesce to form globules, though the globules are never as prominent as they are in fatty infiltration. It represents a more violent or a more prolonged nutrition minus or toxæmia than albuminous degeneration, therefore cells so affected less readily return to the normal.

FATTY INFILTRATION.

Synonym: Lipomatosis.

Nature: Generally physiological, witness adipose tissue; usually physiological in liver.

Causes: Too much fat ingestion; too much ingestion of easily oxidizable substances, such as alcohol. The alcohol is burned and the other food elements are stored up as fat. This includes albumen and carbo-hydrates, which

are converted into fats and stored. Fatty infiltration is a storing up of fat within the cells without any decrease in the amount of albumen in the cell. It may represent the storing of fat brought to the cell as fat, or it may represent fat manufactured by the cell out of albumens and carbo-hydrates. Note differences here from fatty degeneration.

Results histologically: Return to normal; fatty degeneration frequently ensues.

Effects physiologically: Much less than it would seem possible; it interferes but little with the chemistry or the physics of the cells.

Anatomy: Organ markedly increased in size and consistency; edges rounded; very pale; greasy feel.

Microscopic appearance: Signet ring, a central mass of fat that in specimens, as ordinarily prepared, has dissolved away, leaving a clear zone; around this is a rim of compressed protoplasm, and at one side is the nucleus—the signet; protoplasm and nucleus are clear and distinct, unless secondary degenerations have taken place.

Chemistry: See fatty degeneration.

AMYLOID DEGENERATION.

Synonyms: Waxy; lardaceous.

Causes: Prolonged suppuration; syphilis; tuberculosis; leukæmia. It is due to nutrition minus; the elements lacking are not understood.

Results histologically: We do not know that it leads to necrosis; nor do we know that it may disappear and the fibers return to normal; yet there are good reasons for thinking that the latter occurs.

Effects: Impairment of function.

Site: Connective tissues and especially vessel walls; where disease is just beginning, it is to be found in the middle coat of the arteries of small size.

Anatomy: Organ very large with rounded edges; firm; pale; surface glistens. Thin sections made with a parallel bladed knife may show the waxy material. Stain such a section with a mixture of iodine 1, potassium iodine 10, water 100. The waxy areas become mahogany brown, the others a straw yellow.

Microscopic appearance: In the middle coat of the vessel between the muscle fibers; here there is a deposit of this albuminoid substance as a result of a reaction between the cells here

and the plasma; walls thickened; homogeneous, glistening, muscle fibers atrophying; connective tissue cells enclosed by this material are atrophying; epithelial cells not affected by the amyloid process, though it may undergo fatty or other degeneration.

Chemically: Stain sections for five minutes in methyl violet, then for one minute in a saturated watery solution of oxalic acid; wash in water thoroughly, then mount in Farrant's solution. The tissue cells will be stained blue; amyloid will be red. It resists acids and alkalies, is not soluble in alcohol nor water, nor does gastric juice digest it.

Nature of the process: The material is not a starch. It contains nitrogen in about the same proportion as albumens, yet it is not acted upon by acids, alkalies or the gastric juice. It is a mixed infiltration and degeneration; the appearances and all the characteristics are those of an infiltration, but there must be a primary change in both the fibers and in the chemistry of the plasma.

Usual sites: Glomeruli of kidney, capillaries of liver, corpuscles of spleen.

HYALINE DEGENERATION.

Synonym: Vitreous degeneration.

Causes: Nutrition minus.

Locations: In muscles that have been ruptured or overstrained there is always hyaline degeneration in the affected areas. This is especially true after prolonged toxæmias, such as typhoid fever; found here in rectus abdominalis, because of the strain to which it is subjected in changing posture. Found in blood clots shielded from infection; therefore frequent in the ovary and in thrombi. Found in tumors, especially in those of the abdomen; in the thyroid gland in goiter.

Effects physiologically: Loss of function.

Microscopic appearance: Intrinsically it cannot be differentiated from mucoid and from amyloid; all three are hyaline degenerations.

Chemistry: Stains markedly with acid stains, especially oesin.

MUCOID AND COLLOID DEGENERATIONS.

Location: Found in carcinoma in which the epithelium springs from mucus secreting epithelium. In chondromata, lipomata, myxomata, myomata, gliomata and sarcomata; in the walls of glands, such as in the secreting

structure of the stomach; secondarily it involves the fibrous stroma of such structures.

Effects histologically: In the protoplasm of the cell a globule of hyaline material appears. This increases in size until the cell is distended, much as the cell is distended in fatty infiltration. The cell ruptures and the mass becomes an even lake of mucoid material, intersected by fibrous tissue walls.

Microchemistry: It is precipitated as a granular material by acetic acid. It is less firm than is colloid.

GLYCOGEN INFILTRATION.   ·

Synonyms: None.

Cause: Nutrition plus.

Nature: Occurs in the liver and many other localities when too much carbo-hydrates are taken; found especially in diabetes, in which some step in the destruction of carbo-hydrates is interfered with.

Effects physiologically: Cells and fibers are swollen by a clear and homogeneous mass, or by a granular substance arranged in globules.

Microchemistry: Soluble in water; gives the amyloid reaction with iodine, but does not stain blue with sulphuric acid. This in-

filtrate being soluble in water, the section must at no time come in contact with water. Fix, harden, embed, cut, wash in benzine. Alcohol. A mixture of 1 part tr. iodine and 4 parts of absolute alcohol; oil origanum; balsam.

An infiltration may represent nutrition plus. The normal individual cell if in a state of nutrition plus works extra hard and begets its kind. In the infiltrations of nutrition plus the protoplasm of the individual cells is un-affected or even in nutrition minus. It is the general system which is nutrition plus, not the infiltrated cell.

In the degenerations, which all represent nutrition minus, there is a class of affections in which nutrition is entirely at an end. These are called the necroses, and take several names, dependent upon what happens after the cells are dead.

Necrosis in a general way is first to be described. Due to entire cessation of nutrition, because either no food is furnished, or else the protoplasm of the cell is so altered that it is incapable of appropriating food. Therefore frequent causes are:

1.—Thrombus and embolus.
    Angio-sclerosis.
    Pressure.

2.—Burns, scalds, freezing.

Ergot.

Infections.

Nerve lesions.

Effects physiologically: Loss of function.

Microscopical appearance: The nucleus disappears, the protoplasm becomes granular, the cell outlines are lost, a mass of granular material is the sole representative of the tissue.

Chemical reaction: Elements stain with great difficulty.

The area of necrosis is frequently the seat of infection with pus germs; result—suppuration. It frequently is the seat of a deposit of lime salts—calcareous degeneration.

Calcareous degeneration. Microscopical appearance: Opaque; granules and plates. If to a section under the microscope a drop of a mineral acid be added, the granules disappear and bubbles of carbon dioxide accumulate under the cover.

Nature: A combination of fatty acids and acids derived therefrom, with lime basis of the blood and tissue juices.

Most frequent locations: Atheromatous patches in arteris, tumors, old suppurations, such as pleurisies.

Caseation: If from an area of necrosis the fluids absorb, the resulting relatively dry mass is an area of caseation.

Liquefaction: Such a necrosed area or a living area may be acted on by digestive ferments secreted by bacilli, leucocytes, or from other sources so that the protoplasm of the cells and intercellular substance is dissolved in the fluids of the part.

Coagulation necrosis: Necrosis plus coagulation; death in the cells accompanied or followed by coagulation in its protoplasm.

Most frequent site; the pharynx in diphtheria.

Gangrene: Necrosis of a considerable area, with primary or secondary infection.

Causes: Those of necrosis (see above), cold, pressure, arteriosclerosis, or better angiosclerosis, for the sclerosis may be in vessels other than the arteries; nervous diseases; ergot. Infection; several organisms; most frequent bacillus of malignant œdema, bacillus coli communis.

Gross appearance: Organ black, greenish (from decomposing blood) with raised blebs filled with reddish to greenish fluid. Odor may be foul, dependent on infecting germ.

HEALING OF WOUNDS.

In this I will describe the process by which an incised wound in a soft part heals.

The incision severs capillaries, lymphatics, nerve filaments and both epithelial and connective tissue cells.

1. The plasma and blood flow into the rent and coagulate, binding together the two sides of the incision.

2. The portions of the cells cut away from their nuclei die and are absorbed by the exuded leucocytes.

3. The cells irritated, by (a) the direct stimulus of the cut, and (b) the indirect stimulus through the nerves that are hurt—divide by indirect division:

4. These cells and leucocytes wander into the clot.

5. Capillary loops, springing from the capillaries, developing step by step with the cell development, extend into the clot.

6. The gap, being filled to the skin level, the epithelial cells grow over the surface.

Note. The irritation causing the epithelium to proliferate is supplied, as in the case of the underlying tissue, by (1) the direct stimulus of the cut and (2) by the indirect stimulus through the hurt nerves. New cells were being

formed from the beginning. They do not stick until the skin level is reached.

7. The leucocytes carry off any tissue not needed for permanent structure.

8. The connective tissue cells certainly, and the leucocytes possibly, mature into connective tissues.

9. The blood capillaries disappear by (1) contraction of maturing fibers, (2) by endarteritis obliterans.

The above is called healing by first intention. If the plasma does not glue together the surfaces, and if a larger space is to be filled in, the histologic granulations become anatomic, and we term the process healing by second intention. The only difference is in degree.

Healthy granulations are those in which there is a pari passu growth between embryonal blood vessels and young tissue cells.

Foul graulations are those in which there is a loss of relation between growth of embryonal blood vessels and young tissue cells.

The necessity for healing by second intention arises most frequently from infection.

TUMORS.

A tumor is a cystic or solid new growth. They are divided into:

1. Connective tissue tumors.
2. Epithelial tumors.
3. Dermoids.
4. Teratomata.
5. Cysts.

The connective tissue tumors are:

A. Benign—
>   Fibromata.
>   Lipomata.
>   Myxomata.
>   Chondromata.
>   Osteomata.
>   Odontomata.
>   Gliomata.
>   Myomata.
>   Angiomata.
>   Lymphangiomata.
>   And a few less important modifications of some of these.

B. Malignant—
>   Sarcomata.

The epithelial tumors are:

A.   Benign—
       Papillomata.
       Adenomata.
       Neuromata.

B.   Malignant—
       Epitheliomata.
       Carcinomata.

A dermoid is a tumor composed of hair, teeth, etc., developed from an inclusion of some blastic structure in an area abnormal to it. This inclusion is characterized by a tendency to make mature tissues.

A teratoma is developed from a second ovum, acting as a parasite on the host; e. g., a four-legged man or a double-headed calf.

A cyst is a pathological mass of fluid constituents surrounded by a wall.

CAUSE OF TUMORS.

There are two principal theories, neither of of which has been demonstrated.

(1) That tumors, and especially malignant tumors, are due to organisms. These organisms are held to belong to the protozoa or to the yeasts.

(2) That tumors are remnants of fœtal structures or inclusions of post-natal structures that in later life develop.

FIBROMATA.

These can be taken as the basis of connective tissue tumors, both benign and malignant—a tumor composed of white fibrous connective tissue.

Location: Anywhere in the body.

Varieties: Simple fibroma, molluscum fibrosum, keloid, false neuroma endothelioma.

Anatomy: These tumors are generally multiple; they are always incapsulated and benign. They are generally hard, dense, and on cut section are found to be composed of bands of fibers running in various directions.

Histology: The tumor is composed of fibrillated connective tissues, running in various directions, generally in dense bundles; amongst the fibers there are a few spindle-shaped nuclei; there is a comparatively small number of blood vessels, and these have fully matured walls.

Degenerations: Serous, mucoid, fatty—calcification—cyst formation. These tumors are liable to inflammations.

LIPOMATA.

Location: Found anywhere in the body, but more abundant in the subcutaneous tissues; may be multiple, when they are gener-

ally small, or there may be a single large tumor.

Anatomy: The tumors move freely on the underlying structures; generally the skin slips easily over them, though sometimes they are attached to this structure. They are rounded, lobulated, encapsulated, and show as masses of yellow fat with trabeculæ of white fibrous connective tissue.

Histology: That of adipose tissue; connective tissue cells are filled with globules of fat, the protoplasm showing as a ring around the globules; nucleus found as an enlargement at one point of this ring.

Degenerations: Molecular softening, a starvation necrosis, in which the tumor elements break down into granular debris and fatty crystals; calcareous infiltrations subsequent to the first variety of degenerations mentioned. They are subject to inflammation and ulceration.

Lipomata can be considered as bearing the same relation to fibromata that adipose tissue does to ordinary white fibrous tissue.

MYXOMATA.

Tumors made up of branching connective tissue cells, infiltrated with mucoid material.

Location: Found in any part of the body, but more frequently in the nose and in the subcutaneous connective tissue.

Anatomy: These tumors grow slowly; lobulated, encapsulated. From this capsule trabeculæ run into the tumor mass. The spaces between the trabeculæ are filled by a mass of clear, gelatinous material, resembling boiled tapioca. If a small portion of this tumor be immersed in dilute acetic acid, the clear, gelatinous areas become slightly opaque, losing their luster.

Histology: There are bands of fibrous tissue, composed of fibers with a small number of cells. In these bands are matured blood vessels; between the bands are zones, consisting of a comparatively delicate connective tissue reticulum, with spaces filled in with mucin. The individual cells of this reticulum are branched.

Degenerations: Hemorrhage, from rupture of the vessels; ulcerative inflammation.

A myxoma may be said to be a fibroma infiltrated with mucoid substance.

CHONDROMATA.

Location: Periosteum of bones; in the parotid and salivary glands, testicle, skin, mamma.

Anatomy: The growths are not infrequently multiple. They are firm, elastic, rounded, lobulated, with distinct fibrous capsule, trabeculæ running in therefrom. The tumor cuts with a creaky, cartilaginous feeling.

Histology: Between the bands of fibrous tissue there are areas of hyaline matrix, in which are the usual cartilage cells placed in a cartilage cell space. In some of these spaces there are two nuclei.

Degenerations: They are subject to myxomatous or mucoid infiltration; to bone formation; to calcification; to ulcerative inflammation.

OSTEOMATA.

Location: They grow chiefly at points of junction between a bone and cartilage.

Varieties: Eburnated, compact, spongy.

Eburnated osteomata are found always in the vicinity of bone or on the surface of bone. They consist of dense 2 bone, laminated in structure, the layers parallel with the free surface; no Haversian systems.

The compact osteomata are found in bone, and in a good many connective tissue areas entirely separated from bone. The structure is that of normal bone. There is a periosteal covering, and the bone is around Haversian systems.

The spongy osteomata are those in which the Haversian canals are very wide, and comparatively few layers of bone have been deposited by the osteoblasts.

GLYOMATA.

It is doubtful if these should be classed among the connective tissue tumors, since many histologists hold that the neuroglia cells are derived from the epiblast. They are tumors, composed of neuroglia cells.

Anatomy: They are found in the central nervous system; are usually single, sometimes multiple. Encapsulated, gray to reddish in color; frequently distinguished from the brain substance with great difficulty. Sometimes raises the brain substance so as to give the appearance of an hypertrophy of the convolutions. In processes of hardening the tumor structure shrinks from the brain substance, so that it stands out more prominently.

Histology: There is a recticulum of delicate fibers. These fibers are protoplasmic prolongations of small cells characterized by these branching processes. The cells have one or more deeply stained nuclei, and seem to stud the mass of fibrous recticulum. The number of blood vessels is very considerable:

some are young with thin walls; some are old with thick walls; there are usually considerable numbers of large cells thickly studded with golden-brown pigment.

Degenerations: Hæmorrhagic infiltration, from rupture of the vessels; fatty degeneration; starvation necrosis.

MYOMATA.

Two varieties:

(1.) Leiomyomata, composed of non-striated muscle; and

(2.) Rhabdomyomata, composed of striated muscle.

LEIOMYOMATA.

They are by far the more frequent of the two.

Location: Uterus; broad ligament; ovary; gastro-intestinal tract; prostrate gland.

Anatomy: They are generally encapsulated; firm; multiple. Cut section has a banded appearance, bands running in every direction. They vary very greatly in the number of blood vessels; not infrequently they contain so large a number of blood vessels that they give the appearance of angioma.

Histology: The tumor consists of interlacing bundles of involuntary muscle, with

large, rather rounded nuclei. It is difficult
to tell this tumor from fibroma when the tumor is matured.

Degenerations: Mucoid; fatty; necrosis,
followed by calcification; cyst formation; infection.

ANGIOMATA AND LYMPHANGIOMATA.

Angiomata are tumors composed of blood
vessels. Lymphangiomata are tumors composed of lymph vessels.

ANGIOMATA.

Are divided into (1) simple angiomata, in
which the blood vessels are of moderate diameter; and (2) cavernous angiomata, in which
the blood vessels are widely dilated.

Synonyms: Nævus, birth marks.

Location: In the subcutaneous tissue, especially of the face, in the tongue, in the
liver.

Anatomy: An angiomata shows as a plaque
—red in color if the blood is arterial, dark if
venous; very slightly elevated above the surface.

Histology: The tumors are found to be
composed of blood vessels, embedded in
areolar tissue. These blood vessels are of

normal size in simple angioma; in cavernous angioma they consist of lakes, bounded by comparatively thin fibrous tissue walls.

LYMPHANGIOMATA.

Location: In the tongue; in the subcutaneous tissue; in the mucous membrane of the lips.

Anatomy: A pale, pinkish patch, very slightly raised above the surrounding surface.

Macroglossia is lymphangioma of the tongue.

Histology: The tumor is composed of lymph tubes.

SARCOMATA.

Varieties: Round celled, small and large; spindle celled, small and large; myeloid sarcoma; melano sarcoma. We seldom find a sarcoma composed of one variety of cells alone. The tumor generally bears the name of that variety of cell which predominates.

Location: In any organ of the body.

Nature: Malignant, malignancy being in the following order: Melano sarcoma, round celled, spindle celled, fibro sarcoma.

Etiology: Not known. They present a perfect picture of connective tissue reaction

to irritation. There exists but little doubt but that they are parasitic in origin.

General characteristics: They have no capsule, except where they have developed in an organ with a capsule, in which event the capsule is not theirs, but is the capsule of the organ. They are more frequent in young people. They are richly supplied with vessels, the vessels being in the same state of immaturity as the cell. They grow rapidly, infiltrate the surrounding structures, causing degeneration and absorption of the elements of the part invaded. They spread by blood vessels, and in consequence metastases are found in the first set of capillaries through which the blood passes after leaving the tumor. They are composed of connective tissue cells, which begin as round cells, with an inherent tendency to form fibers. They are malignant just in the same proportion as this tendency is interfered with; not that the round cell is in itself more malignant than the spindle cell or the fiber, but that the cause which produces them in so great rapidity and with such abnormality that they do not have time or disposition to proceed beyond round cells, would be violently injurious to other centers,

for but a small part of the effects of sarcoma are local, the larger part are constitutional.

ROUND CELLED SARCOMATA.

Anatomy: The tumor is very soft, generally rounded, but without a capsule. On section it has an even pink appearance, with small red or brown hæmorrhagic patches.

Histology: The tumor is composed of round cells, usually small, sometimes large, with a single nucleus, and with a minimum amount of intercellular substance. In the midst of the round cells are blood vessels whose only wall consists of a single layer of elongated cells.

MELANO SARCOMA.

Anatomy: These tumors are small, rarely larger than one inch in diameter. They are dark in color, frequently almost black; the color is comparatively uniform. They are soft in consistency, have no capsule; they form metastases while yet the tumor is almost microscopic in size.

Histology: The cells are round cells, generally larger than in the small round celled sarcomata. There are many spindles. They are filled with rather coarse pigment granules;

but these pigment granules do not give the color reactions of melanin.

Location: Choroid coat of the eye; the skin; the suprarenal capsules; they very frequently form a secondary growth in the liver.

SPINDLE CELLED SARCOMATA.

Location: In any connective tissue structures; metastases are not so frequent as in round celled sarcomata—the lung is the most frequent seat of secondary growth, liver second in frequency.

Malignancy: Less malignant than round celled sarcomata.

Anatomy: May have reached considerable size. There may be some external condensation of fibers, resembling a capsule. On cut section the tumor is moderately firm and fleshy in appearance.

Histology: There is an abundance of spindle cells, either small or large; among these spindle cells are large numbers of blood vessels with embryonal walls, that is, walls composed of a single layer of spindle cells arranged end to end.

GIANT CELLED SARCOMATA.

Synonym: Myeloid sarcomata; epulis.

Location: Found especially in connection with bone and periosteum.

Anatomy: The tumor grows with only moderate rapidity; it very frequently has an apparent capsule; it is moderately firm and elastic, pinkish in color; it is irregular both in color and in consistency. Not infrequently islands of bone are found in its midst.

Histology: There is a great abundance of round and spindle cells and embryonal blood vessels, and among these are large, irregular masses of protoplasm, with multiple nuclei. These cells resemble osteoclasts, and give the appearance of cells set in nests.

This tumor in malignancy varies within wide limits.

EPITHELIAL TUMORS.

BENIGN EPITHELIAL GROWTHS.

PAPILLOMATA.

Varieties: Corns, warts, vegetations, horns.

General characteristics: There is a central stalk of fibrous tissue covered by epithelium. This epithelium may be piled up in an indefinite number of layers, but its basement membrane is unbroken, and the lower germinating layers of epithelium show no tendency to grow into the underlying structures.

ADENOMA.

These are new developments of glands in which the epithelium arranges itself in a normal fashion. The glands are always functionally inactive. The epithelium is set on a basement membrane, and shows no disposition to invade this basement membrane. These tumors are on the border line of malignancy, and no hard and fast line of benignancy can be drawn.

NEUROMATA.

Two varieties: (1) Composed of nerve fibrils, and (2) composed of ganglion cells. These tumors are rare.

MALIGNANT EPITHELIAL GROWTHS.

Varieties: Springing from squamous covering epithelium, called epitheliomata; and growing from glandular epithelium, called carcinomata.

General considerations: Carcinomata are rare except in points where mechanical irritation is frequent. They are more frequent in maturer life. They spread by lymphatics alone, except late in their history, when general carcinosis is possible. Generally speaking, they are more malignant than sarcomata, and the hypoblastic carcinomata are more malignant than those of epiblastic origin.

Malignant adenomata, called carcinomata, differ from benign adenomata in that they are never encapsulated, properly speaking. They are never polypoid or pedunculated; and the epithelium not only fills the glandular acini, but it breaks through the basement membrane, and extends, as more or less regular gland tubes, into the surrounding structures.

EPITHELIOMATA.

Location: The lips, the tongue, the anus, the penis, the vagina and cervix of the uterus, the skin and the subcutaneous tissues.

Method of spreading: These tumors stick to the lymphatic channels very much more closely and invade the blood channels with much more reluctancy than any of the other malignant growths.

Anatomy: They may present either one of two forms.

1. Fungus, in which there are rich vegetations projecting above the surface. These vegetations bleed readily, and are the seat of a foul, sanious discharge.

2. Flat ulcerating form in which the tumor level is below that of the surrounding tissues.

Histology: At the margin of the malignant area, the normal epithelium of the surface can be seen growing into the underlying tissue, in bands or fingers, or columns of epithelial cells. These cells are dividing actively. The finger shape is given by the shape of the lymph tube in which they are contained. In places, in which there is less resistance on the part of the invaded tissue, the cells are gathered together in nests. The cells in these nests are generally concentrically af-

ranged. The connective tissue between the lymph tubes, sometimes called the alveolar walls, may be normal, or they may be the seat of a simple inflammation; inflammatory cells, and sometimes giant cells, are found in the midst of the epithelial cell masses. The blood vessels are in the connective tissue walls.

Degenerations: (1) pearls; the cells of which these tumors are formed are subject to keratin degeneration; and, therefore, in their new locations, as they become old, or are subjected to pressure, they form nests of keratin, called epithelial pearls. Pearls are not found except in cells derived from areas that are prone to keratin transformation. (2) Secondary infection and round cell inflammation.

Infection: Neighboring lymph glands.

CARCINOMATA.

The shape of the epithelial cells and their arrangement within the alveoli, depends (1) upon the epithelium and arrangement in the structure from which the carcinoma grew, and, (2) upon the tissues into which it grows; for example, a carcinoma springing from columnar epithelium arranged in a glandular arrangement is very prone to retain both the shape of the epithelial cell and its arrange-

ment. Such a carcinoma, growing from the mucous membrane of the stomach in the submucosa, will be distinctly glandular; but, traversing the muscular coats, we will see columns of epithelial cells. These take the glandular arrangement upon reaching the serous surface. These tumors, growing from epithelium which normally has a tendency to dip into the underlying structures, more easily invade those structures than do the epitheliomata. They are, therefore, more malignant.

Anatomy: The tumors have no capsule and no pedicle; they are closely attached to the surrounding tissues. On cut section they are generally soft, pink, with trabeculæ of fibrous tissue mapping them off into areas. There may be ulceration.

Histology: The walls, called alveoli, are composed of fibrous tissue, that may or not be filled with roud cells of inflammation. In this fibrous tissue stroma are the blood vessels of the cancer. The epithelial cells may be arranged as fairly regular columnar epithelial gland tubes, or they may be nests of epithelial cells of any shape or size.

Degenerations: They are subject to the same degenerations as the epithelium in the

locality from which the tumor sprung; e. g..
(1) carcinomata springing from the gastro-
intestinal tract, therefore areas of mucus-se-
creting cells. are prone to colloid degeneration;
(2) infections; (3) ulcerations.

DERMOIDS.

Location: In the ovary; testicle, subcutaneous tissue, especially of the median line:
along the lines of fœtal union; e. g., around the
branchial clefts. They are generally cysts,
containing sebaceous matter, skin, hair, nails,
teeth, mucous membrane.

CYSTS.

These are divided into:

1. Retention cysts; cysts formed in a gland
duct in which the lumen of the duct has become occluded; e. g., ranulæ, ovules of Naboth.

2. Secretion cysts, those taking place in
ductless gland structures as a result of loss
of relation between secretion and absorption,
e. g., cysts of the thyroid gland; bursæ.

3. Degeneration cysts, ensuing by degeneration and liquefaction, e. g., around bullets
and other foreign bodies, an area of infarct;
cold abscesses.

THE RESPIRATORY APPARATUS.

SOME POINTS IN HISTOLOGY.

Nose; portions of the pharynx; larynx; trachea; bronchial tubes, lung substance and the pleura. All, with the exception of the pleura, are tubes, certain parts that do special work have a special arrangement. The tube consists of an intima, a media, and an adventitia. The intima is especially well developed, and is imperfectly divided into a mucosa and submucosa. The media is divided into a longitudinal and a circular layer. The adventitia in some places contains cartilage plates.

From within out, the layers are:

1. A single layer of ciliated epithelial cells, columnar in type.
2. A basement membrane. ⎫
3. A mucosa. ⎬ Mucosa.
4. A muscularis mucosa. ⎭
5. A submucosa.
6. Inner longitudinal muscle. ⎫ Media.
7. Outer circular muscle. ⎭
8. A fibrous tissue coat.—Adventitia.

In the fœtus there is nothing to the lungs but these tubes. When at birth, air is forcibly inhaled, the tubes are stretched into sacs, called air spaces and foyers, called infundibuli.

In the air sacs the necessities are for a free interchange of gases between the air spaces and the blood in the capillaries.

The walls of air vesicle then are:

1. Stretched, thin, epithelial scales.

2. Connective tissue, white fibrous and yellow elastic.

3. A connective tissue blood vessel wall.

4. A layer of endothelial cells.

These are the four layers, all thin and delicate, which gases have to traverse. The bronchial tubes break into tubes of constantly diminishing size.

As the force of suction is applied to the air cells and as one bronchial tube supplies numberless air cells, it is very necessary that the bronchial tubes should not collapse, so that cartilage plates are located in their fibrous coats.

Bronchi less than 1 mm.—terminal bronchi structure.

1. Single layer of ciliated columnar epithelial cells.

2. Mucosa, elastic fibers, a few muscle fibers, and lymphoid tissue.

A terminal bronchiole and its vesicles is termed a lobule.

The ligaments of the lungs—bands of white fibrous and yellow elastic tissue, run from the root of the lung to the pleura.

There is a double set of arteries:

1. Pulmonary arteries.
2. Bronchial arteries.

Lymphatic tissue is very abundant. Most of the channels begin in the air cell walls, follow the walls of the bronchial tubes and filter through the bronchial glands at the root of the lung. Others (1) run in the septa, (2) a few near the pleura drain to that membrane.

Pleura:

1. A layer of large flat endothelial cells with stomata between.
2. White fibrous tissue, yellow elastic tissue, and some nonstriated muscle.

This connective tissue, its vessels and its lymphatics, communicate slightly with the underlying lung. The amount of communication is in the order in which the tissues are named.

PNEUMONIAS.

The term pneumonia is used in lieu of pneumonitis, to indicate inflammation of the

lung. It includes all of the inflammatory processes, acute and chronic, in the interstitial tissue and air vesicles. It does not apply to inflammation of the pleura or bronchi.

As the lungs have no chemistry aside from the chemistry of their own nutrition they are not prone to degenerations. They are lowly organized, being simply a tryst for the gases borne in the air current on the one hand, and in the blood current on the other. These inflammations are therefore nearly always germ inflammations.

Acute pneumonias:

Lobar, exudative in type.

Lobular, productive in type. (Exudation less prominent.)

Abscess, destructive in type.

Gangrene, destructive in type with a secondary infection with saprophytes.

Hypostatic, mildly exudative.

Chronic pneumonias:

Interstitial, productive in type.

A group due to physical irritation, as anthracosis in coal miners; silicosis in sand workers; siderosis in metal workers.

Tubercular.

Syphilitic.

Heart disease.

(A) ACUTE INFLAMMATIONS.

LOBAR PNEUMONIA.

Synonyms: Croupous, pneumonia; lung fever.

Cause: In order of frequency—diplococcus of Fraenkel, bacillus of Friedlander, streptococcus, staphylococcus; always microbic in origin.

Nature of process: Exudative, productive inflammation, spending its force on the vasomotor apparatus; a type of exudative inflammation.

Anatomy: Usually involves the lower lobe of one lung; may involve a middle or upper lobe, usually most marked on lower and more dependent surface. Lung swollen and shows imprint of ribs; injection of overlying pleura with effusion of some fluid, which may or may not be coagulated. Lung bright red, dark red, mottled gray and red, or gray, according to the stage of the process. If all alveoli are filled, it sinks in water. In any event it floats deep in the water. Heavy "cuts" resistant. Pressure causes a bloody froth to exude from

the cut bronchioles. The consistency is about even everywhere in the affected lobe. The bronchial and mediastinal glands are swollen.

Philosophy of the process: Pneumococcus secretes its toxine, which irritates vasomotor nerves; vessels dilate, fluids exude, white and red cells go out freely. The foreign material goes into the alveoli as the areas of least resistance. The epithelial plates of the air cells are washed away, the connective tissue cells proliferate. The white and red cell producers are stimulated into compensatory activity. The absorbed toxine acts on the heat centers, causing fever; on the sensory centers, causing malaise, headaches, etc.; on the heart centers, causing fast pulse; on the respiratory centers, causing hastened respiration; on the liver and kidney cells it acts as a stimulant to function, or, the irritation becoming more violent, inflammatory degeneration ensues with lessening of function.

Congestion and exudation: Until the plasma coagulates, the stage is called congestion and exudation.

In this stage from the cut surface the exudate can be squeezed until the lung collapses completely.

Red hepatization: When the exudate has coagulated, the stage is called hepatization, and its first substage is red hepatization; red because of the red cells in the exudate; hepatization, because the filled lobule looks like the liver lobule. The air vesicles are in varying degree filled with a skein of delicate fibrin filaments, holding in its meshes red cells, white cells, inflammatory cells, and epithelial cells. The packing is close, and the alveolar wall is made out with dfficulty. The vessels of the alveolar wall can be seen filled with blood, and its connective tissue is filled with proliferating cells.

Gray hepatization: The next substage is called gray hepatization. It is the first step toward liquefaction. The appearance starts as an irregular distributed marking, which gradually diffuse from multiple foci, until there is a moderately even color. The gray is due to the dark reduced hæmoglobin and the whiter fibrin, leucocytes, and inflammatory cells. The serum has either been coughed up, or has been absorbed through the vessels and lymphatics. The fibrin is beginning to liquefy from the ferment of the germs and of the leucocytes. The air vesicles are not so full; a thin, clear area begins

to bound the exudate, the wall shows plainer, and its vessels are more full. When the process of liquefaction has been completed and the exudate is again fluid, as it was in the stage called exudation, we call it resolution.

Resolution: The fibrin is liquid, the cells (red, white and inflammatory) have undergone fatty degeneration and liquefaction. The vessels are approaching their regular size, the cells are ceasing their division. The lymphatics are filled with debris; pigment is abundant. This result has been brought about by an anti-pneumotoxine.

Sequelæ: This is the type of result in the cases which recover. Remember it is a violent toxæmia, and not a local affection; that it is caused by a germ that is just short of sufficient virulence to cause necrosis in this lowly organized tissue. It may on the one hand cause necrosis, abscess or gangrene; on the other hand, it may be less irritating than usual, when the reactionary processes are not operative to the same degree, liquefaction does not ensue, but into the clot within the alveoli connective tissue grows from the walls, giving a nonresolving, chronic interstitial pneumonia. These lungs are prone to tubercular infection.

BRONCHO PNEUMONIA.

Synonyms: Lobular pneumonia, catarrhal pneumonia, pneumonia of childhood, capillary bronchitis.

Causes: An irritant, milder in type than those causing lobular pneumonia. Generally the streptococcus and staphylococcus, perhaps also the organism of pertussis, measles and scarlet fever. The number of organisms which may be pathogenic here is large. The irritant enters by the bronchial tube.

Nature of the process: A bronchitis is usually the starting point. The cause of this bronchitis either gets into the deeper layers of the bronchi, from which it extends by lymphatic continuity to the alveolar walls surrounding, or else it extends to the air vesicle by force of the air current. This last is not as considerable a factor as it would seem, as in the smaller tubes exchange of gases is not by currents. The flow of lymph and blood is from the alveolar to the bronchial wall, so we expect very few of the cases of bronchitis to cause broncho-pneumonia.

Histology: It involves a lobule, and has a bronchiole as its center. In this tube the epithelium is degenerating; the mucosa and submucosa are infiltrated with inflammatory

cells, which are piling over the bronchial glands and destroying the regularity of the individual layers. The alveoli contiguous are filled with the products of exudative and proliferative inflammations, fibrin, white, red and connective tissue cells; the alveolar walls are filled with inflammatory cells. In the outer zone the poisoning is less severe, and the alveoli are filled with epithelial and connective tissue cells; the alveolar walls are thickened by connective tissue inflammatory cells—a productive inflammation.

Such an inflammation has a lessened tendency toward resolution as compared with lobar pneumonia, because (1) the less severe infection does not produce as large an amount of a curative product, and (2) there is more connective tissue proliferation in the alveolar walls and in the deeper layers of the bronchial tube.

Anatomy: The lung is usually irregularly mottled. It is diffusely œdematous, with here and there wedges of denser lobules that are solid. If it is a surface lobule, it projects above the surface, thus being distinguished from atelectasis, in which the solid area is sunken. From the tubes muco - purulent material is squeezed. An extensive bronchi-

tis may eventuate in an extensive pneumonia, when you get a lung much resembling lobar pneumonia. Look closely, especially near the periphery of the lobe, for evidences of lobulation.

Complicating pneumonias are generally lobular in type; they may be lobar.

HYPOSTATIC PNEUMONIA.

Etiology: Two elements.

1. Loss of relation between the power exerted by the right ventricle on the one hand, and friction, gravity and other forces to be overcome by this power on the other. This element causes venous congestion and an exudate, consisting of much water and salts, little plasma, few leucocytes, fewer red cells.

2. Infection of the area of poor nutrition.

The factors in the first are weakening of the power of the heart, or impediment to the return of blood. So the question rapidly gets back to the universal question of lowered resistance and consequent infection. The germs are of about the same limitations as broncho-pneumonia. The channels of invasion are the bronchial tubes and the vascular channels, carrying infection from the original site, e. g., pus germs from the typhoid ulcer.

Anatomy: The dependent part of the lung is dark, full of blood, œdematous, with scattered patches of broncho-pneumonia. On cut section the bloody froth squeezes out until the lung is collapsed, except in the islands of inflammation. As there are these several factors, the variations in appearance are almost limitless.

ABSCESS.

(1) Pyæmic.

(2) Secondary to lobar or broncho-pneumonia.

Pyæmic: Usually multiple, small, widely distributed, but generally near the surface.

Secondary: Larger, single, or few in number. May be anywhere, but more frequent in the upper lobe. They may not, though they generally do, communicate with a bronchial tube.

Routes of infection: (1) Blood current, (2) bronchi.

Cause: Any organism that either is usually or could under these circumstances become pus producing.

Histology: In each the same; a central zone of pus; next a layer of degenerated cells that do not take any stain, mixed with deeply

stained leucocytes; next a layer of granulation tissue, water soaked, consisting of embryonal vessels, leucocytes, and connective tissue cells; next an older layer of cells varying from round to matured connective tissue, according to the age of the process. Partial obliteration of the air vesicles, general thickening of the alveolar walls. The lymphatics carry an excessive amount of pigment; swelling of the glands.

Cure takes place by (1) destruction of the organisms, or habituation of the tissues to them so that their toxine is no longer irritating; and (2) growth of tissue from the walls until the cavity is obliterated.

GANGRENE.

Cause: Infection with a gas producing saprophyte.

Nutrition is usually cut off from the lung by thrombus, embolus or aneurism; this, however, is not necessary.

Recognized by the unaided senses by (1) odor, (2) color; bacteriologically by organism isolated; microscopically the findings are those of necrosis.

(B) CHRONIC INFLAMMATIONS.

CHRONIC INTERSTITIAL PNEUMONIA.

Synonyms: Substantial emphysema; Corrigan's lung; cirrhotic lung.

Definition: A chronic inflammation of interstitial tissue of the lung, that is not due to disease of the heart, the tubercle bacillus, the syphilis bacillus, actinomycosis hominis, or the mechanical irritants as coal dust, stone dust, or what not.

Etiology: It is due to a mild irritation long continued. It is caused in frequency in the following order: Asthma, broncho-pneumonia, lobar pneumonia, pleurisy, collapse.

Philosophy of the process: There is a new growth of connective tissue, most of which is at any given time fully matured. There is always thickening of the pleura and of the bronchial wall, and one or the other of them assumes unusual prominence, according to the area of origin of the disease. All interstitial processes are uneven processes— that is to say, the amount of aveolar thicken-

ing will be greater in some zones than in others. The tendency of inflammatory connective tissue to contract is to be borne in mind. Therefore some of the tubes and the air vesicles will be obliterated, or nearly so, by the connective tissue overgrowth and contraction, and others will be dilated even to cyst formation. The epithelium of the vesicles springs from cubical epithelium; so under the disturbed conditions it again becomes cubical.

Disturbances in circulation result in extravasations of blood; disturbed nutrition results in loss of cilia from epithelium, so that pigmentation is usually more marked than it is in health.

Anatomy: The lung is small, pale, firm, with a very thick pleura. If it is collapsed it is found next the vertebræ, reaching to or almost to, the diaphragm on its posterior surface. On section it is pale, tough, resistant, sometimes gritty.

Histology: Microscopically we find connective tissue bands with spindle shaped nuclei scattered here and there. These bands surround openings of irregular size and shape. The smallest of these are occupied by small masses of round epithelial cells, apparently

lying loose in the space, but in a good state of nutrition, as evidenced by the clearness of detail and the vividness of the staining. Other openings are much more readily recognized as alveoli. These are lined by a single layer of cubical epithelial cells, generally very regularly arranged. In still other areas the only change is in a thickening of the alveolar wall to about twice its regular diameter, together with some tendency to a cuboid shape in the epithelium. The greatest thickening of the connective tissue is in those areas where the conditions are most inviting, and this is near those broad connective tissue bands that radiate from the root of the lung to the pleura, and are sometimes called the ligaments of the lungs. The next greatest overgrowth is beneath the pleura.

Ultimate effects: Eventually the lung will almost entirely lose its capacity as a sac. At this time it is largely indifferent to all forms of infection.

PNEUMONIA OF HEART DISEASE.

Synonyms: Brown induration of the lungs; mechanical hyperæmia; brown œdema.

Cause: Long continued disease in the mitral and aortic valves.

Philosophy of the process: The leak in the heart valves increases the pressure in the pulmonary veins. This is compensated for in a measure by the yellow elastic tissue in the walls of the veins, but here the elastic fibers are far fewer than in the arteries; the increased pressure extends to the capillaries: the capillaries are tortuous and loosely surrounded. They dilate both in diameter and in length—cirsoid aneurism. This causes them to project, knob-like, into the air vesicles; the obstruction from above causes a slowing of the current. This means decreased nutrition and a prolonged bathing, both in their own leucomaines and in the leucomaines from the other tissues of the body. The result of this mild irritation long continued is an overgrowth of connective tissue—alveolar. The epithelium becomes cubical or round and proliferates. These make hæmorrhage by rhexis and diapedesis easy, and so there is an excess of pigment.

Anatomy: The lung is brown, somewhat small, heavy; "cuts" with difficulty; much dark blood exudes. It may be, and frequently is, œdematous.

Histology: There is a moderate increase in connective tissue, which is moderately

well matured, though not as fully as in other forms of interstitial inflammation. The vessels are seen projecting as globular knobs on each side of the alveolar walls; many of the alveoli are filled with large round epithelial cells containing reddish brown pigment.

ANTHRACOSIS, SIDEROSIS, SILICOSIS.

Synonyms: Coal miners' phthisis; scissors-grinders' phthisis; stonemasons' phthisis; lithicosis; chalicosis.

Etiology: Chemically inert, but physically irritating particles of coal, metal, stone or what not are deposited on the bronchial walls beyond the zone of cilia, and in the air vesicles themselves. Nature wisely provides that no air currents shall go beyond the latitude of cilia, but nevertheless some particles fall in the forbidden territory. They admirably fill the requirements of a mild irritation long continued.

Philosophy of the process: The irritating particles are carried into the lymph channels to the alveolar walls, and from there to those of the septa. They set up productive inflammation; as most of the lymph channels are perivascular, changes rapidly involve the vessels; this connective tissue contracts; nutri-

tion is shut off and necrosis from starvation ensues.

Anatomy: The pleura is thickened, and there are adhesions of varying toughness. The lung is very black when the irritant is coal dust, less so when it is otherwise. There is increase in weight and in resistance. It "cuts" tough and often gritty. Here and there are nodules reaching considerable size. On cut section the center is yellow detritus; this may be calcified. The periphery is dense, laminated; it merges into the surrounding tissues. The glands are large and black, not only the glands of the root, but those throughout the septa. The septa are more than usually prominent.

Histology: In the center of these nodules is a mass of tissue detritus mingled with some mineral material. Around this is a zone of denser connective tissue; outside this a zone of newly proliferating connective tissue with an abundance of nuclei and round cells. In these zones there is evidence of diffuse arteritis, thickening of the adventitia and media, and active proliferation of the cells of the intima. All of the alveolar walls are

thickened. Some of the alveolar epithelium
is normal in position and in shape; some is
cubical or flat; some is loose in the vesicle;
some of the cells contain pigment.

TUBERCULOSIS AND PHTHISIS.

Under the head of tuberculosis we will treat those affections in which the tubercle bacillus is alone operative; under phthisis those cases in which there is engrafted on the lungs a second infection.

Then tuberculosis is an interstitial inflammation with a strong tendency to become localized; a nodular interstitial pneumonia due to the tubercle bacillus. Phthisis is tuberculosis plus pneumonia.

TUBERCULOSIS.

Varieties: Subacute and chronic.

Etiology: Tubercle bacillus.

Channel of infection: Blood current.

Philosophy of the process: The tubercle bacillus lodges in a capillary. It secretes its toxin. This toxin is a mild irritant. The local tissues are stimulated into activity; leucocytes rapidly wander to the local area. If the irritant is rather severe, the central cells immediately surrounding the bacillus die; those further away develop into fibers; some

form giant cells, if the process is not too
acute. This intermingled developed and developing mass of cells, leucocytes and connective tissue cells give the reticulated appearance that is so suggestive of tuberculosis.
If the bacilli are not very virulent, they are
either circumscribed by connective tissue ci-
catrices, or else they are destroyed by phagocytes and the tubercular process is at an end.
The mass of inflammatory tissue may be absorbed entirely, though this is unusual. It
may become calcified. It usually remains as
an old cicatricial mass with rarely caseated
foci. The inflammatory masses necessarily
involve nerve endings. This irritation, which
in nerves of sensation would be intrepreted
by pain, in nerves of sight by a light picture,
is in this locality interpreted by cough; cough
means some mechanical injury to the bronchial tubes. So a light bronchitis may com-
plicate the tubercular process.

Anatomy: Such a lung is usually moderately congested and mildly œdematous. Here
and there are multiple small nodules, rather
more frequently found in the lower lobe than
in the upper. They vary from a size too small
to be seen with the naked eye, to the size of
a pea. In color they are gray to pearly gray,

when growing; yellowish, when breaking
down.

Histology: We may have:

1.   Miliary tubercles, typical in character
In the center is a giant cell, about ten times
the diameter of the ordinary cell, with as
many as twenty nuclei arranged around the
periphery of the protoplasm. This protoplasm
may be quite granular. Tubercle bacilli can
frequently be stained within them, though
when they pick up the bacillus, the bacillus
very promptly loses its power to take up a
stain. Frequently the border of the giant
cell seems to shade into the surrounding intercellular substance; frequently from it prolongations seem to run to the contiguous
fibrillæ. Around this will be a zone of mixed
leucocytes, connective tissue cells and fibers.
The contiguous blood vessels show some inflammation of the endarterium, but much
more inflammation of the adventitia. The
variations from this type usually consist in the
following:

1.   The center is caseated.

2.   The tubercle is made up of round cells
and leucocytes alone.

In addition to the tubercle, in its vicinity
there will be seen a somewhat even thickening of the alveolar walls.

PHTHISIS.

Phthisis is tuberculosis plus pneumonia. If one or the other or both conjointly are violent processes, the lesion rapidly ends life, and is known as acute phthisis. If these factors are less violent and the reaction thereto is less forceful, the result is common chronic phthisis or ulcerative phthisis. If these factors are still less forceful, destruction of tissue is less prominent, maturing of tissue is more prominent, and fibroid phthisis is the result. Between these three there are no lines of demarkation, and there are cases that are placed in different categories according to the individuality of the observer.

ACUTE PHTHISIS.

Etiology: The tubercle bacillus and any of the other organisms. The most frequent are staphylococcus, streptococcus, pyocyaneus, bacilluscoli communis, pneumococcus. For be it known that the lesions of the tubercle bacillus are productive; they are but mildly destructive, but they render infection with other organisms very easy.

Philosophy of the process: The tubercular lesion is produced as in the other case. Owing to the lack of time giant cell systems

are not prominent. Owing to the complicating organisms, destructive processes are more prominent. The channel of infection is through the air routes and the lymphatics; the route of the secondary infection is through the bronchial tube. As the elements that enter into the causation are multiple, the variations from the type become more prominent. For intsance, the accidental placing near to or far away from a bronchial tube makes a great difference in the time of secondary infection, and therefore in the prominence of destruction.

Anatomy: The pleura is usually thickened; there are fresh adhesions, especially at the apex; the lung is solid, perhaps entirely, perhaps in a lobe. It is red and heavy. Here and there are yellow patches; these are more prominent at the apex. Cut sections may show within their patches a cavity communicating with a bronchial tube, and containing some pus, or it may be merely a mass of cheesy material with a less distinct wall than in the first instance. The near neighborhood of the cavity will be solid; as we go farther away, it becomes progressively more open. From the tubes, pus and mucus exude on pressure.

Histology: The center of the nodule shows only amorphous material. In a single microscopical section we may find multiple foci of degeneration. Around the patch of breaking down is an area of round cells, leucocytes and fibrous tissue mesh; vessels can be made out with difficulty here. Further out the condition merges into a simple alveolar thickening. Here the vessels show plainly. Here the air vesicles are filled, not by overgrowth of the connective tissue of the alveolar wall as is the case in the tubercular area, but by pneumonic products, fibrin filaments, white cells, red cells, connective tissue and epithelial cells.

COMMON CHRONIC PHTHISIS.

Synonyms: Consumption; ulcerative phthisis.

Cause: Tubercle bacillus plus other organisms.

Channel of infection: Bronchi and lymph vessels.

Philosophy of the process: Same as in acute phthisis, except that the processes have more time to develop. The vessels are better spared than in any of the other inflammations of this group (syphilis, sarcoma,

actinomycosis); the lesions are usually periarteritis. Endarteritis is less marked.

Anatomy: The process is usually most
marked at the apex of one lung, though both
may be involved. The pleura is thickened,
and tubercles are the rule rather than the exception. There are old adhesions over the
zone of inflammation and sometimes elsewhere. The cavity may be obliterated;
effusion, clear or bloody or purulent, may be
present. The lung shows hard nodules,
wedge-shaped, separated by patches of the
consistency of simple inflammation. Lymph
glands and septa are involved. On section
multiple, ragged walled cavities are seen.
These are in a measure filled with pus that
may be colored and odored, dependent upon
the germs growing there. Connective tissue
bands and blood vessels may stretch across,
unsupported; around the cavities, in the walls,
and further away are fibrous nodules, some of
which are yellow and caseated, others gray
shading off to pink. Between these nodules
are zones presenting the appearance either of
lobar or broncho pneumonia.

Histology: A caseous area, surrounded by
mingled cells and fibers; giant cell systems
are here more prominent than in any other
form of tuberculosis. There is a large quan-

tity of old matured dense connective tissue. In this tissue is an abundance of pigment in tracts that were once lymphatic channels. Blood vessels of small size can be demonstrated with difficulty. Those of larger size have their adventitia swollen and thickened, or ulcerated if secondary infection is operating on them. The walls of the bronchi are the seat of tubercular nodules that extend into the lumen, or ulcerate and leave cavities communicating with the tube. The old scar tissue contracting in many places destroys the relations of the parts. The alveolar walls in the vicinity of the nodules are thickened to twice the normal size. The alveoli are filled with fibrin, white and red cells, detritus, epithelial cells.

Cure takes place from (1) defeat of the bacillus and its companions by (a) discharge, (b) phagocytic action, (c) exclusion from maturing connective tissues.

Death ensues from toxæmia.

SYPHILIS.

Synonym: Lues.

Etiology: Possibly the syphilis bacillus of Lustgarten.

Philosophy of the process: A leucocyte and

connective tissue resistance to the toxins of the germ.

The disease is rare in the lungs. It gives a lesion which is similar to tuberculosis, except that endarteritis is much more prominent. The channel of infection here is the blood vessel, and this in part accounts for the prominence of the lesion of the intima.

The other inflammations of this character to which the lungs are subject are:

Actinomycocsis, due to the actinomyces hominis, and giving small millet-seed-yellow masses in the midst of the inflammation and in the pus.

Glanders, due to the bacillus mallei. Giving small nodules, miliary and multiple if the infection be from the blood, and frequently single and ulcerated if from the air passages. When miliary and degenerated they may be yellow, or stained the color of any pigment that happens to be present.

TUMORS OF THE LUNGS.

The primary tumors found in the lungs are lipoma, osteoma, fibroma, chondroma, cylindrical celled carcinoma, sarcoma.

The secondary tumors are much the more frequent, because the lungs present the first set of capillaries that a malignant fragment

would encounter after leaving its site of origin. As sarcoma contains so many wall-less vessels, and as they frequently spring from the intima of veins, they constitute the bulk of secondary tumors.

PARASITES OF THE LUNGS.

All of the vegetable parasites that can be carried by the air or by the blood current.

Amongst the animal parasites: The amœba coli, hydatids, filaria bronchialis and cysticercus cellulosæ.

ACUTE BRONCHITIS.

Etiology: First, bacterial, influenza bacillus, pus cocci, pneumococci, the germ of measles, smallpox, scarlet fever. Second, inhalation of gases, powders, steam.

Nature of the process: An acute exudative, productive inflammation. It is much more liable to involve the smaller bronchi and the lung substance in children than in adults.

Anatomy: The lung is congested and œdematous. On squeezing a section serum oozes from the substance and muco-purulent material comes from the bronchi. On laying open a bronchus its wall is seen to be thickened. The mucosa is especially thickened. It is covered by tenacious muco-pus.

When this is removed the membrane has lost its luster. It is red and uneven.

Histology: Epithelial surface. The epithelial cells are irregular in shape; in many places they have fallen away entirely. Many are in a state of cloudy swelling. Among the epithelial cells are leucocytes, red cells and round cells of inflammation. The fibers of the basement membrane are separated by new cells and leucocytes. The inner fibrous, muscular and outer fibrous coat are closely packed with round cells. The intensity of the process is less as we go outward. At the periphery it extends along the lymphatics.

Sequelæ: It may undergo resolution. It may go on to the chronic disorder. It may eventuate in broncho pneumonia.

Atelectasis: Collapse of the lung. Due to (1) imperfect expansion immediately after birth. (2) Penetrating wounds of the pleura and chest walls. (3) Plugging as in bronchitis.

Bronchiectasis: Dilatation of bronchial wall, from any cause, either within the wall or within the fibrous structures attached to it.

Emphysema: Overdilation of the air vesicles. Found in old people in heart disease, asthma, whooping cough, chronic interstitial pneumonia, pleurisy of the other side.

It is not infrequently compensatory, that is to say, that when the respiratory capacity of one lung is decreased the other increases *pari passu*. The term emphysema is also applied to that condition in which from rupture of vesicle or bronchial wall air is loose in the midst of the tissues.

PLEURITIS.

Synonyms: Pleurisy, empyema.

Varieties: Dry pleurisy, pleurisy with effusion, pleurisy with adhesions, pleurisy with formation of fibrin, suppurating pleurisy, tubercular pleurisy:

Nature of the process: Pleurisy is always an exudative, productive inflammation. The fluid seeks the cavity as the area of least resistance. The pleura has large capacity for absorption. If the amount of exudation is within the capacity of the pleura for absorption, no fluids accumulate, the inflammatory cells develop into fibers; the pleura is thickened—dry pleurisy.

If the amount of effusion is large, it accumulates as a straw colored fluid in the dependent parts of the pleura; proliferation of the inflamed area causes thickening; pleurisy with effusion. If coagulation occurs in the exudation, we have pleurisy with the

formation of fibrin. If this fibrin glues together adjacent parts of the pleura, then connective tissues and capillary blood vessels
grow into the coagulated fibrin. This continues until a band of fibrous tissue unites
the "glued" parts—pleurisy with adhesions.

If infection of the pleura has been with
pus germs the process becomes suppurative;
the pleural cavity becomes a true abscess
cavity—empyema. Tubercular pleurisy does
not differ from tuberculosis elsewhere.

Basic histology of pleurisy: The epithelial cells that cover the inflamed area swell
and fall off. Inflammatory cells are massed
among the connective tissue fibers. These
cells pile up on the surface. Capillary blood
vessels grow from older vessels, tunneling
their way among the new cells. The process
ends by the new cells maturing into fibers,
which fibers contract. The new vessels disappear by (1) contraction of fiber, (2) endarteritis obliterans. The area is covered by
(1) epithelial cells growing from the neighboring epithelium, or (2) the cavity is obliterated by union of its parietal and visceral
layers, or (3) the superficial connective tissue
cells are condensed and flattened as in large
scars in other localities.

CIRCULATORY SYSTEM.

HEART, ARTERIES, CAPILLARIES, VEINS, LYMPHATICS.

The whole contents of the blood current have not made the double circuit until the lymphatics have emptied their contents. The whole constitutes a tube. This tube has three coats, an intima, a media and an adventitia. There is one part of the tube that has to do much muscular work; its muscularis is well developed; we call this muscularis the myocardium. There is another part of the tube that must permit of no leaking, and must receive the intermittent force and convert it into an even force; it is the aorta; hence it is dense, little muscular, but very elastic from an abundance of yellow elastic tissue. There is another part that must permit an interchange of gasses and liquids between, within and without; its wall must be thin; it is the capillary, with a wall consisting of a single layer of endothelial cells and a little loose connective tissue. There is another part that must change its size in order to regulate pres-

sure and nutrition; this is the arteriole with prominent circular muscular fibers. There is another part which must not leak, nor stretch much, nor permit the blood to flow back; this is the vein, with the intima loose and picked up into folds—valves. In all of them no blood soaks in further than the intima, so a separate set of vessels is provided to nourish the other coats; those in the heart are called coronary arteries, in the vessels the vasa vasorum.

The heart is inclosed in a sac similar in its anatomy and in its histology to the pleura. This sac is called the pericardium. Underneath this is a layer of loose connective tissue that usually contains fat. This is the epicardium or adventitia. Under this is a mass of muscle fibers, running in every direction, separated by bands of fibrous tissue continuous with the fibrous tissue of the epicardium. These fibers are involuntary, striated, branched. In the embryonal state, and in certain of the lower animals, the protoplasm is granular and there are no striæ; striation begins at the poles and in different animals approaches the center in varying degree—in man according to the degree of disturbance of normal processes of repair. The cor-

onary arteries and their capillaries radiate in the epicardium and myocardium, and in a small measure in the endocardium. The inner layer consists of white fibrous and yellow elastic tissue, covered by a single layer of endothelial cells, just as in a serous membrane. Valves are made by a picking up of this endocardium.

Arteries: A loose adventitia of white fibrous and yellow elastic connective tissue; in this are the larger branches of the vasa vasorum. Next comes the media, mostly muscle fibers —nonstriated, arranged circularly, some longitudinally—and some yellow elastic and some white fibrous connective tissue, in which are the smaller branches of the vasa vasorum. Internally the intima with a thin layer of yellow elastic tissue, called the inner elastic lamina, forming its outer border; then a mixture of white fibrous and yellow elastic tissue, covered or lined by a single layer of endothelial cells.   .

The parenchyma of the heart is its muscle fibers; muscle work is the physical expression of chemical equation; therefore the heart is a highly differentiated organ. It is prone to inflammatory changes. In its physiological nutritional changes, such as hypertrophy and

atrophy, are prominent. It is subject to many of the degenerations and to various tumor growths, both secondary and primary. Systemic infection is prone to attack its lining coat, though its other layers are very free from them, as the coronary arteries are given off at right angles to the direction of the main current and solid particles, such as bacteria, travel with the main direction of the current.

The degenerations to which the heart is subject are: cloudy swelling, fatty and hyaline degenerations, myomalacia, and those which are common to every tissue and present no structural peculiarities, necrosis and calcification.

CLOUDY SWELLING.

Synonyms: Albuminous degeneration, acute parenchymatous degeneration.

Cause: Toxæmias from organic poisons, e. g., typhoid fever, pneumonia, diphtheria, septicæmia, burns; inorganic poisons, e. g., phosphorus, iodoform.

Philosophy of the process: The protoplasm of the muscle fiber is a delicate semisolid. These poisons change its chemistry so that certain elements precipitate as solid granules and the protoplasm takes up water

from the intercellular substance. In the same line of chemical change is fatty degeneration, and if the process proceeds slowly, fatty change soon ensues. If the process is more rapid, there ensues a granular degeneration, called in this area myomalacia.

Anatomy: The muscular wall is soft and friable. The deep red flesh color is lost, and a dirty gray, boiled appearance is substituted.

Histology: The fibers are swollen, finely granular; the striæ obscure or absent; nuclei obscured or cannot be seen. Fresh unstained specimens mounted in salt solution, or acetic acid run under the cover, will show fibers normal in appearance. Ether and osmic acid will not affect the granules.

FATTY DEGENERATION.

Cause: Organic poisons longer continued as those of phthisis, pernicious anæmia, leucocythæmia, Addison's disease, septicæmia; inorganic poisons longer continued, as phosphorus, arsenic, alcohol; nutrition minus, slowly progressing, as in sclerosis of the coronary arteries.

Philosophy of the process: The precipitated albumen granules, having lost their

chemical relations to the balance of the protoplasm, enter the next stage of slow death, fatty metamorphosis. In sclerosis, nutrition minus destroys the balance between waste and repair, and the lower protoplasm (fat) is substituted for the higher. It is impossible to explain why the process should be an uneven one.

Anatomy: The heart is flabby and friable. The cavities are dilated. The fatty changes show as white, creamy, smooth patches, usually beginning under endocardium, and especially in the musculi papillares and columnæ carneæ. A thrush-breast, or streak of lean and streak of fat appearance here, is characteristic of the earlier stages.

Histology: There may be slight increase in the number of round cells in the connective tissue, especially around the blood vessels. This, however, is not prominent. The muscle fibers are swollen slightly. Their striæ are absent or indistinct, especially around the center of the fiber. The nucleus is obscured or unseen. The globules are larger and more refractile than in cloudy swelling. If under cover of a piece mounted unstained you run ether, the granules disappear, contrary to what you find in cloudy

swelling.   Acetic acid, run under cover, has
no effect.   Osmic acid stains the globules jet
black and renders them brittle.

Finale.   The condition may be cleared up
and return to the normal if the cause is removed; or, it may result in myomalacia,
aneurism, rupture, or interstitial myocarditis.

FATTY INFILTRATION.

This condition does not belong in the same
category as fatty degeneration, yet it will be
treated here.

Synonyms: Fatty overgrowth of the heart;
lipomatosis; adipose heart.

Cause: General obesity; alcohol.

Philosophy of the process: From surcharg-
ing the blood with hydrocarbons and carbo-
hydrates, some fat is stored in many connective tissue cells for future use.   One of the
most constant sites is the loose tissue over
the myocardium.   So long as it is limited to
this area, it is of little consequence; but
when it begins to be deposited in the connective tissue septa that run down into the
myocardium, it, on the one hand, places the
muscle fibers at a disadvantage, and, on the
other, causes fatty degeneration.

Anatomy: The heart is large, covered by

a heavy layer of fat. Lines of pale fat extend down into the myocardium. The ventricles are apt to be dilated, and the muscle flabby for the same reason that every muscle in such a subject is flabby. Such subjects are prone to the arterio-sclerosis and atheromas.

Histology: In the connective tissue are the typical appearances of adipose tissue. In specimens hardened in alcohol, you see large clear circles, signet ring shaped, being a ring of protoplasm and the nucleus crowded to one corner. If the specimen was hardened with osmic acid, these globules are black and opaque. In advanced cases these globules are found in the septa and in the connective tissue bundles between the muscle fibers.

HYALINE DEGENERATION.

Causes: Prolonged toxæmias of typhoid.

Philosophy of the process: The change is in the muscle fiber. The supposition is that by reason of some strain, when the fiber is weak, as in cloudy swelling, it ruptures, whereupon the protoplasm undergoes this change into hyaline material.

Histology: The affected fibers have lost their striated appearance, are homogeneous, refractile and shiny. They stain with eosin.

MYOMALACIA.

Nature of process: A form of necrosis.

PRODUCTIVE MYOCARDITIS.

This lesion is an accompaniment of endocarditis and pericarditis. It is limited to a
zone near the one of these in which it starts.
To illustrate: Beneath the endocardium is a
small area in which there is cloudy swelling
of the muscle fibers and round cell proliferation in the connective tissue with some dilatation of the vessels, stasis and exudation.

Inflammations of the myocardium are productive and suppurative; neither is prominent.

SUPPURATIVE.

The route of infection is the blood vessels.
As the coronaries come off at right angles, it
is rare. It may be quite diffused, or localized,
forming abscess.

CHRONIC MYOCARDITIS.

Cause: In the great majority of instances,
sclerosis of the coronary arteries.

Philosophy of the process: Nutrition
minus, and overgrowth of connective tissue.

Anatomy: There is usually marked evidence of endocarditis and endarteritis. The

coronary arteries have thickened walls; they are stiff, patulous, and often atheromatous; many of their branches are obliterated. There are usually present milk-white fatty patches underneath the endocardium, especially near the columnæ carneæ. Here and there, generally in the left ventricular wall other than the septum, there is a white and brown streaking. These areas are firmer than normal, though the heart wall as a whole is apt to be fatty.

Histology: There is a marked increase in the connective tissue. This tissue is usually old, fibrillated: It is most marked around the vessels and lymphatics and in the connective tissue septa. At its margin the tissue is younger, and in its loops are seen muscle fibers—some degenerating, some in a good state of preservation. Thickening of the arterial walls is much in evidence.

ENDOCARDITIS.

(1) Acute; (2) simple, and (3) ulcerative. The only difference between these processes is a difference of degree. If the process produces tissue, which dies only from nutrition minus, we call it simple endocarditis; if death of the produced tissue, and of some old tissue as well, is due to active enzymes, we call it ulcerative.

Cause: The most frequent cause of the first and second is rheumatism, gout, scarlatina; the third is due to organisms that locate on the endocardium. The more frequent of these are the streptococci, staphylococci, gonococci and pyocyanei. It seems probable that most any pathogenic germ can induce the trouble.

Philosophy of the process: As a result of irritation from toxines, connective tissue proliferates. The process is a productive inflammation, and as the endocardium is free from vessels, it is an excellent illustration of productive inflammation. As a result of proliferation, an endocardial mass is formed, which projects into the lumen. The histology and the chemistry of the endothelium are both changed; behind the eminence there is a slowing of the current; a coagulum forms; into this connective tissue may grow from the endocardium, and it is then known as a vegetation. Some of these vegetations fracture, and the remnants are swept away to be stopped, and known as emboli. The tissue is not well nourished, for its food must come by omosis; therefore it dies—necrosis. Lime salts from the blood are deposited in the masses of detritus—calcification. The pul-

taceous mass is known as atheroma. Some of these patches empty into the blood current, leaving an ulcer. If the process is ulcerative, clotting is earlier. The germs multiply on the clot; they liquefy it; it fractures easily. The remnants, full of germs, are swept away, to set up the process in new areas. Ulceration is much more prominent.

Anatomy: The endocardium may be somewhat more succulent than normal; this is more liable to be appreciable over the valves. Near the free margins of the mitral and aortic valves will be seen a row of small, semi-transparent, friable warts. Some of these may have broken off, leaving ragged ulcers behind. In the ulcerative form the vegetations will be softer, will pull away easier, and more patches of ulceration will be seen.

Histology: In the coagulum we find leucocytes, some red cells, and fibrin in layers that show some tendency to be alternate. In the clot next the endocardium, connective tissue round cells are appearing. Deeper down we have a mass of inflammatory connective tissue and leucocytes, spindle and round cells. Here embryonal vessels, derived from the myocardium, can sometimes be made out. In patches there is evidence of

granular degeneration, necrosis, or ulceration.

CHRONIC ENDOCARDITIS.

Causes: Rheumatism; gout; acute endocarditis.

Philosophy of the process: The difference between this and the acute process is the change that time makes in inflammatory connective tissue.

Anatomy: The heart is apt to be fatty and sclerotic. The walls are nearly always either dilated or hypertrophied, or both dilated and hypertrophied. The process is usually in evidence in the aorta, and not infrequently in the coronaries. The vegetations are on the side of contact; that is, on the ventricular side of the aorta, and on the auricular side of the mitral. The vegetations are firmer and more adherent; the valves are sometimes glutinated at their edges; sometimes they are scarred, thickened, and so retracted that they cannot close the orifice. They may be the seat of calcareous plaques, and these plaques are frequently covered by endothelium, and frequently are bare. There are erosions and curdy masses here and there.

Histology: The histology is that of chronic

productive inflammation, with marked tendency to necrosis and calcifications.

Effects: Stenosis, or leaking; embolus; angina; hypertrophy and dilatation; connective tissue overgrowth in the liver and lungs.

BROWN ATROPHY OF THE HEART.

Synonym: Pigmentary degeneration.

Cause: Old age; phthisis; anæmia; Addison's disease.

Philosophy of the process: In the fœtus, and in certain of the lower animals, the heart protoplasm is a granular mass without transverse striations, or with striation only apparent at the extremities of the fibers. Under these conditions of perturbed nutrition, there is this exhibition of embryonal return. The pigment is not from the blood; it is from the fiber.

Anatomy: The heart is small, flabby, dark brown in color. Held on the tips of the fingers, it falls over the hand. It may be changed somewhat by associated fatty changes.

Histology: The ends of the heart fiber are normal. Around the nucleus, in the area called "Schultze's corpuscle," there is marked granularity and pigmentation. The pigment is golden yellow. The area is far in excess

of the size of that found in the normal heart. Between the muscle fibers there is an overgrowth of connective tissue.

HYPERTROPHY OF THE HEART.

Cause: When from any cause there is increase in the work demanded of the heart, it hypertrophies.

Hypertrophies are (1) true, and (2) false.

A true hypertrophy is an increase in the size of each fiber. A false hypertrophy is an increase in the number of fibers. The increased work causes increase in both the size and the number of fibers. It is prone to be followed by atrophy, when dilatation ensues; or, hypertrophy and atrophy may be associated, as when the heart increases in size and pari passu with the increase in size and number of the corpuscles, there is atrophy of certain fibers next to the cavity of the ventricle.

SCLEROSIS OF THE CORONARY ARTERIES.

The coronary arteries are prone to both endarteritis deformans and obliterans. These processes present no peculiarities in this locality. But there are certain effects on the heart muscle, and its contained nerves, that are worthy of note.

Effects: Angina pectoris; neuralgia from nutrition minus; fatty degeneration; sclerosis; interstitial myocarditis; abscess from infection of a branch with pus germs.

Myomalacia—nutrition rapidly minus.

Aneurism—nutrition minus over a limited area.

Rupture—nutrition minus over a limited area, muscular power retained in other areas, and an extraordinary compressing of the contained blood.

INFLAMMATIONS IN ARTERIES.

We have inflammations of the coats of arteries—periarteritis, mesarteritis and endarteritis. The inflammations that are of greatest practical interest are the forms of endarteritis. These are endarteritis deformans and obliterans, the difference between them being that endarteritis obliterans is a diffuse endarteritis, and the other is in plaques. Obliterans has a growth of capillaries into the new tissue of the intima from the media; deformans has none. For this reason, deformans is much more subject to regressive phenomena, atheroma, calcification.

Inflammation of the intima is very prone to involve the media as well.

ENDARTERITIS OBLITERANS.

Process by which obliteration of the inflamed capillaries takes place.

Cause: Continuation of a mild irritation, as syphilis, alcohol.

This is the condition found in arterio-sclerosis. It is a precursor of, or associated with sclerosis in the kidneys, liver, cord, brain, etc.

Philosophy of the process: The entire vessel is mildly irritated. There is a productive inflammation of the connective tissue of the intima and inner layers of the media. The capillaries of the vasa-vasorum send off shoots into the intima, which proliferate indefinitely, or until the space is occupied, the lumen is obliterated.

Anatomy: The vessel wall is thickened evenly; there are seldom any patches of atheroma; the intima is usually preserved.

Histology: There is a layer of young, flattened cells next the intima; outside of this a region of young connective tissue cells, in which young capillaries are appearing.

The inner elastic lamina is considerably broken up by the new connective tissue and vessel proliferation. The media may be thinned; connective tissue is proliferating

here. There is usually some inflammation in the adventitia.

ENDARTERITIS DEFORMANS.

Synonym: Atheroma.

Cause: Found especially in the vessels of old people. It is a nutritional disease. It is most frequent due to leucomaines 'or ptomaines that are very mild in their capacity for irritation.

Philosophy of the process: The irritation is applied to scattered spots, so it is an inflammation in plaques. As it is a pure connective tissue proliferation without any growth of vessels, it is much more prone to degeneration, called atheroma. As the nutrition of the intima comes largely from the blood current, it is the layers next the inner elastic lamina that first begin to die. The intima is preserved for a considerable time, and this is a very wise provision.

Anatomy: There are patches placed irregularly along the walls of the vessel, sometimes on one side and sometimes on the other. They are pink or pearly when young, but soon become curdy, then yellowish. They are at first resistant to the knife, then become gritty. The patches are by prefer-

ence located at the points of greatest friction, and especially around the orifices of branches. It is a disease to which the aorta, the coronaries and the cerebral arteries are very prone. Owing to the irregular location of the plaques, the blood current runs from side to side, first near one bank and then near the other. At first over the plaques can be seen the shining endothelium; later this is lost. The calcareous mass may be covered by blood clot. Sometimes the mass of degenerated tissue has dropped out, and a ragged, denuded patch, called an atheromatous ulcer, is left.

Histology: There is a proliferation of connective tissue, especially in the intima, so that this layer is many times its normal thickness. Its inner layer, which was concave, may now be convex. Under the endothelium there appear between the laminæ of fibers layers of cells. This process continues indefinitely. The landmark of this area, the wavy elastic lamina, is seen to separate the media from the connective tissue proliferation. In these streaks of cells, and especially in those next the inner elastic lamina, granular and fatty degeneration begins to appear; then the fibers become granular and fatty.

These areas become dark and translucent if they have been brought to the microscope without change. If hydrochloric acid is run under the cover the granules disappear and bubbles of carbon dioxide appear.

Effects: Thrombosis, embolism, a slight tendency to aneurism and varicosities, rupture.

MESARTERIUM.

The middle coat of the artery is subject to chronic inflammation, to inflammatory degeneration, to fatty degeneration, to calcification, and to waxy degeneration.

In old people the media of the middle sized arteries become so calcified as to give a lime tube. This especially is true of the arteries of the brain.

As the media is the strong coat, to inflammatory or degenerative changes in it are due most of the forms of aneurism.

The media of small vessels, and the remnant of the media and adventitia of still smaller vessels, is the seat of waxy degeneration. There is a prior change in the muscle fiber that makes possible the soaking with modified plasma.

In such a vessel the lumen is encroached upon, but the chief expansion seems to be

outward. Microscopically we see a broad, shiny, waxy band, interspersed with spindle shaped connective tissue and rod shaped muscle nuclei. The percentage of nuclei is small. (For staining see chapter on degenerations.)

The adventitia also inflames, but its inflammations are peculiar to, and connected with, the surrounding connective tissue rather than with the structures of the deeper layers. It is a very wise provision that in no location in the body is it as nearly possible for pathological processes, in structures so close together, to be so dissociated.

Aneurisms: Aneurisms are divided into two classes, true and false.

True aneurisms are localized dilatations of the vessel wall, the dilated area being made up of at least one coat of the vessel.

False aneurisms are simply accessory to the vessels, and have as their walls the surrounding tissue or inflammatory new tissue.

The true aneurisms are divided into:

1. Sacculated—in which there has been a localized weakening of the vessel wall; this is usually in the media, sometimes in the adventitia. The point dilates; the more it dilates the greater the pressure in its direc-

tion.   Its walls from without in are adventitia
(media usually absent), intima, layers of fibrin
in process of organization, layers of fresh
fibrin, and blood cells.

2.   Cylindrical and fusiform—in which the
entire periphery bulges out.   The walls are
made up of intima and adventitia; clotting is
much rarer.   It is given one or the other
name, dependent on its shape.

3.   Dissecting—in which there is a rupture
in the intima, and the blood dissects its way
between the layers of the vessel wall.

4.   Miliary—are usually found on the cerebral vessels.   They are sacculated, and their
name comes from their size.   They are generally multiple, and frequently are found in
enormous numbers.

5.   Cirsoid—in which there is an increase
in the breadth and length of the arteries;
they become tortuous;· the condition approaches closely to angioma.   In the veins it
finds a similar condition in varicose veins.

False aneurisms: In these there is a rupture, or several ruptures, of the vessel walls;
these ruptures become permanent.   The
blood forces its way until the surrounding
tissues are resistant enough to circumscribe
it.   If the blood clots, it forms a hæmatoma.

Varicose aneurisms—are true or false aneurisms, opening directly into a vein. The vein here markedly dilates, because its walls are not arranged with a view to resist direct arterial pressure.

VEINS.

The veins are subject to all inflammations and tumor growths that affect the arteries. They are not nearly so subject to intima changes, etc. The tendency to sarcoma-growth in their walls is the most striking tendency in the tumor line. Their tendency to inflame in infectious conditions (typhoid fever, puerperal fever, septicæmia, milk leg with the attendant clotting) is always to be borne in mind.

VARICOSE VEINS.

Synonym: Varix.

Philosophy of the process: The condition is found only in those regions in which the veins that are habitually under heavy gravity pressure are unsupported by the surrounding tissues. Such veins are those of the rectum (piles), the spermatic vein (varicocele), and the leg.

Anatomy: They are tortuous, firm, with

irregular dilatations, and frequently patches of calcification. The normal valves are generally not in evidence.

Histology: There is a new growth of connective tissue in every coat of the vein. The muscle fibers, especially in the stretched areas, are not in evidence. There is usually some necrosis and calcification, especially in those layers of the intima that are next the media.

SOME POINTS IN THE HISTOLOGY OF THE GASTRO-INTESTINAL TRACT.

This tract is a tube. The stomach is a dilatation in the tube. Its intima is divided into two layers, the mucosa and the submucosa, and the separation, which is somewhat indistinct, is by the muscularis muscosa. The intima is thrown into longitudinal folds by muscular contraction. In addition to the folds, which embrace both layers of the intima, the epithelium dips in to form two sets of glands. The epithelium is columnar. The peptic glands, most abundant near the fundus, are straight tubes with two sets of cells, one columnar, lining the lumen; and another, large, round, outside of the columnar layer. The pyloric glands are compound, wavy, and show a disposition to go below the muscularis. The mucosa and the submucosa are connective tissue structures, with many blood vessels, and a large amount of lymph tissue. The most important of the stomach's functions is its motor function; so its muscle layer is most prominent. It is in three lay-

ers, circular, longitudinal and oblique. The adventitia is of little importance.

DISEASES OF THE STOMACH.

1. Acute gastritis.
2. Subacute gastritis.
3. Chronic gastritis—atrophic gastritis.
4. Round ulcer.
5. Cancer.

In discussing stomach conditions it is to be borne in mind that the stomach remains in contact with the gastric juice after death, and that therefore punctures, holes, loss of mucosa etc., may be present, independently of pathological processes. The stomach is a large viscus in which substances remain for some hours, therefore violent irritants show their effects markedly here. It is not distinctively an absorptive organ unless the substance is very volatile. The tissues by which poisons are destroyed or by which they leave the body will be more affected by them than will be organs by which they enter, other things being equal.

ACUTE GASTRITIS.

Cause: Violent irritants of any kind: organic, as ptomaines, tyrotoxicon, decayed

meats; inorganic, as mineral acids, arsenic, phosphorus, etc.

Philosophy of the process: Similar to acute bronchitis, except that there is greater irritation, therefore greater hæmorrhage and stasis of blood.

Anatomy: The mucous surface is covered by mucus, or shreds of mucous membrane if the process is violent, as in poisoning by mineral acids. The mucosa is swollen and irregular. Twigs of injected vessels stand out prominently. The injection on the peritoneal surface is apparent.

Histology: There is abundant small, round cell infiltration of the mucosa, submucosa and of the connective tissue between the muscle fibers. The blood vessels are distended and around them the inflammatory connective tissue proliferation is most marked. The epithelium of the surface and of the glands is swollen, granular and shows either fatty or mucous granules. In places it is falling away.

SUBACUTE GASTRITIS.

Synonyms: Adenomatous gastritis; gastritis glandularis.

Cause: An irritation milder than the one just mentioned, e. g., alcohol.

Philosophy of the process: The position of the process is not well determined. There is an overgrowth of lymphoid tissue and of gland tubes, very similar to that found in endometritis. The gland tubes are lined by epithelium that rapidly becomes mucus secreting. Either as a cause or an effect the muscular coat atrophies. Dilatation takes place and the process is indefinitely continued. More dilatation, more fermentation; therefore more irritation and more adenomatous growth.

Anatomy: The stomach is dilated. The mucosa is greatly thickened; in places it is polypoid; in places it is apparently ulcerated. The muscularis is thickened.

Histology: The mucosa is made up of a mass of round cells, actively proliferating; among the round cells are very irregular gland tubes, the epithelium of which is swollen, granular and oftentimes lying loose in the tubes. The muscularis mucosa is not apparent. The mucous overgrowth impinges on the muscular layers; the muscle layers show some degenerating fibers.

Effects: The effect is a continued secretion of mucus, continued fermentation, growing dilatation, fatty and cirrhotic liver.

ATROPHIC GASTRITIS.

Synonym: Cirrhosis of the stomach.

Philosophy of the process: The inflammatory cells mature; the matured connective tissue contracts, and so obliterates the gastric tubules; it in places causes degeneration of the muscularis.

Anatomy: The stomach is thin-walled and dilated, and may contain a large quantity of clear water or watery secretion, containing some mucus. The mucous surface is irregular; in places it is wholly fibrous, in others polypoid. This tendency to polypoid arrangement is very prominent in any mucous membrane that is bathed in moisture and continuously irritated. ·

Histology: There is an abundance of dense, laminated connective tissue in the mucosa and submucosa. The epithelium is either rounded, irregular in shape or absent. The glands are small in size, and with fairly regular epithelial cells, or else they are cystic, in which event the epithelium is very irregular. This sclerosis extends into the space between the muscular fibers, so they are undergoing pressure atrophy also.

ROUND ULCER OF THE STOMACH.

Synonyms: Solitary ulcer; perforating ulcer; ulcus ventriculi.

Causes: Unknown.

Philosophy of the process: The theory is, there is an embolus, or else an arteritis blocking a branch of the gastric artery. This area, deprived of its nourishment, is digested by the gastric juice. There is a minimum amount of inflammatory reaction in the vicinity of the ulceration; therefore, the particular area must either be subjected to peculiar irritation, or else the tissues must have lost their capacity for resistance in a peculiar way.

Anatomy: The stomach, as a whole, looks very natural. In the great majority of cases the ulcer is found on the posterior surface, or the lesser curvature; the fundus and the cardiac end are nearly always spared. It occurs in women more frequently than in men, and in young people more frequently than in old. It frequently heals. The ulcer has a punched-out appearance. There is little elevation of its edges. Its mucous extremity is the larger extremity. Sometimes it "shelves" as it passes through successive layers of stomach wall. On the peritoneal surface there is often evidence of local peritonitis, and sometimes

the liver, diaphragm, or any adjacent structure, is so closely bound to the stomach as to form a bottom for the ulcer.

Histology: There is little to be seen. In the vicinity of the punched-out area there is a small amount of round cell proliferation. Its striking peculiarity is this negativeness.

DEGENERATIONS.

The stomach is subject to few degenerations beyond the degeneration of the glandular structures into mucous glands.

TUMOR GROWTHS.

The most important of the tumors of the stomach are carcinomata. Carcinoma of the stomach is usually primary in that organ. It is located by preference near the pyloric extremity.

Anatomy: The new growth may present one of two peculiarities; it may be diffused throughout the stomach wall without nodules, or it may produce nodular growths that project into the lumen of the stomach. The first variety has much less tendency to ulceration than has the second. The stomach is usually dilated. The pylorus is contracted, or it may **be widely patulous. There is considerable**

secondary gastritis. There is evidence of extension to the liver, to the diaphragm, to the omentum, mesenteric glands.

Histology: The carcinoma is always of the columnar celled type. There is extension of the epithelium through the basement membrane. In the mucosa and submucosa the epithelial cells attempt to arrange themselves in glands; some of these are easily recognizable as such; some as simple alveoli. While the glands are derived from glandular epithelium, many of them lose their shape, and become simple indifferent epithelium. This epithelium is growing actively. In the muscular layers the epithelium is seen to extend as long, narrow ribbons, one or two cells in width. These are lymph channels, filled. On the peritoneal surface, the epithelium again breaks out into greater activity. There is usually considerable round cell proliferation, and leucocyte invasion in the connective tissue of carcinoma of the stomach.

SMALL INTESTINES.

The small intestine consists of three layers. The most important is the intima. It consists of a mucosa and a submucosa, separated by a muscularis mucosa. The mucosa is thrown

into transverse folds, called valvulæ conniventes. In addition it has normal polypoid growths, called villi. The epithelium is columnar. The glands are simple tubular glands, except in the region of the duodenum, where there is an additional set of duodenal glands that run into the submucosa. The lymphoid tissue is abundant everywhere. It is gathered together in solitary follicles throughout the entire tract. In places, especially in the ileum, there are aggregations of these follicles, called Peyer's patches.

The media is divided into two considerable muscle layers, the inner circular and outer longitudinal layer.

The adventitia is of minor importance.

The peculiarities of the smaller intestine, as distinguished from the stomach, are:

Its transverse folds.

Its villi.

The absence of glands with marginal cells (peptic).

The lesser prominence of the muscle.

The greater prominence of the lymphoid structures.

ACUTE ENTERITIS.

Anatomy: The intestine is intensely injected, especially on the mucous surface. The

color is red. dark red, or brown. There may be injection of the overlying peritoneum. The mucosa is swollen, soft, and covered by thick mucus. This appearance is to be distinguished from post-mortem appearances. There may be some swelling of the adjacent mesenteric glands.

Histology: There is great piling up of the round cells of the mucosa and submucosa. The muscularis mucosa is overrun by these cells. · Here and there are scattered glands. There is no epithelium on the surface, or only a few scattered cells. Amongst the cells are some islands of extravasated blood. There may be round cell proliferation between the bands of muscle fibers of the muscular layers.

TYPHOID INTESTINE.

Synonyms: Enteric fever; dothienteric fever.

Cause: The bacillus typhosus.

Philosophy of the process: The bacillus enters the lymphatics of the intestine, and is carried to the lymph glands, solitary and agminated. Its toxin produces an inflammation. The irritated tissue is destroyed. The bacillus, multiplying in the deeper structures, the inflammatory and destructive process

continues. The gland being destroyed, the poison travels through the muscular coat into the peritoneal, and up to the lymphatic glands. The intestine is in direct continuity with the outside world; therefore the intestine is constantly loaded with germs, pathogenic and otherwise. Through this abraded surface these organisms secure entrance, giving rise to secondary infections of various kinds. To the toxæmiæ are due the cloudy swelling of the liver, kidney and heart, the fever, the rapid pulse and respiration, and the other neuralgias. Perforation is frequently prevented by localized peritonitis. Hæmorrhage is due to ulceration into a vessel in the submucosa or on the peritoneal surface.

Anatomy: The intestine is the seat of an enteritis, which is usually rather mild and diffuse. In the early stages the solitary glands and Peyer's patches are swollen and stand out above the intestinal surface. Later these present themselves as oval ulcers, generally on the side away from the mesenteric attachment. These ulcers have ragged, overhanging edges. There is thickening of the edges in the vicinity of the ulcer. Over the outside there is some local peritonitis. Lymphatic bands, indurated, can be traced to

the neighboring swollen glands. Later those of the patches that did not ulcerate show as shaven beard areas, a streaking of white around small islands of black. The name is descriptive. The glands that ulcerated show as smooth, grayish scars.

Histology: The surrounding tissue shows typical, violent inflammation; round cells pile up over small remnants of epithelial glands; farther away the inflammatory process can be seen extending along lymphatics and in perivascular areas.

TUBERCULOSIS OF THE INTESTINE.

We may have a tubercular peritonitis, in which the tubercles are over the intestinal wall. We have tuberculosis beginning in the mucosa, and this process infecting the peritoneum. When the peritoneum has been infected, either from the blood current or the sexual apparatus, that is, when the infection is from a source other than the intestine, it does not usually ulcerate into the intestine, though it may be productive of diarrhœa. The nerves of the intestine pressed on are apt to give interpretation to irritation in this way.

TUBERCULAR ULCER.

Cause: The tubercle bacillus.

Philosophy of the process: Location generally takes place in the glands; irritation, proliferation. Around each cluster of bacilli there is a nodule of tuberculosis. These necrose, become infected, ulcerate; the ulceration extends irregularly from one nodule to another. The ulceration seldom perforates but the gland being destroyed, tubercle bacilli can spread to the peritoneal surface and thence to the mesenteric glands.

Anatomy: The ulcer is worm-eaten; in its walls tubercular nodules may be apparent; in its bottom tubercular nodules can be felt; over its peritoneal surface there appear tubercular nodules, and the lymphatics can be plainly seen and felt as solid cords.

Histology: There is thickening of the mucosa and submucosa that make up the ulcer wall. They are fairly well covered with epithelium; here are seen tubercular nodules and some show giant cells.

LARGE INTESTINE.

Histology: The large intestine differs from the small in that

1. It has no villi—the fæcal contents are becoming solid.

2. It has no Peyer's patches; the solitary follicles are larger.

3. Its longitudinal muscular fibers are not continuous over the circumference, but are gathered together in bands. It is to this that is due the puckering of the large intestine.

4. More of the glands are mucous glands.

Acute proctitis does not differ in any particular from acute disease elsewhere in the intestine. The gross anatomy and the minute anatomy are the same. It is the seat of a croupous inflammation in which the exuded plasma coagulates on the surface and in the substance of the mucosa and fibrinous casts of the bowels are evacuated. The histology is the same as that of diphtheria in the pharynx or larynx.

ACUTE PROCTITIS.

Synonyms: Dysentery; bloody flux.

Etiology: All kinds of organisms.

Nature of the process: The nature of the diseased process is dependent upon the nature of the infection. It may be what is termed catarrhal, when we have the surface covered by mucus and serous exudate, the epithelial cells, some proliferating and some undergoing mucous degeneration. The blood vessels are

moderately injected, and the mucosa and sub-mucosa contain a few round cells.

In more violent cases, the epithelium is de-generating and falling away, the mucosa and submucosa violently filled with inflammatory cells and exudation products.

In most cases extravasation of red cells is a very prominent feature. In some cases both the mucosa and submucosa may be black and gangrenous.

AMŒBIC COLITIS.

Etiology: The amœba coli.

Nature of the process: The disease is gen-erally subacute. The amœba coli is found most abundant in the submucosa. Here it causes a destructive inflammation. Therefore the markedly overhanging edges of the ulcers. From the colon it is sometimes transported to the liver, where it causes solitary abscess.

Anatomy: The mucosa is swollen, red. There are irregular ulcers in its surface. These have ragged, overhanging edges. Sometimes considerable areas of mucosa can be lifted from its deeper attachments.

Histology: There is moderate increase in the subepithelial mucosa. In places the mu-

cosa is ulcerated away. There is found violent round cell inflammation in the submucosa. The organism, larger than an epithelial cell, can be seen in the mucosa, but it is far more prominent and abundant in the lymph spaces of the submucosa. There may be moderate inflammation in the muscularis and the serosa.

CHRONIC COLITIS.

Other forms of chronic colitis are mucous colitis, follicular colitis.

Mucous colitis: A very moderate inflammatory degeneration, mucous in type, limited to the epithelial structures of the colon. It is characterized by the presence in the stools of mucous casts of the bowel. These casts are molds of the bowel and consist of masses of epithelial cells in a state of marked mucous degeneration. The cells remaining attached to the basement membrane are dividing.

FOLLICULAR COLITIS.

Anatomy: The mucosa is generally not markedly injected. Here and there over its surface are enlarged solitary follicles that project into the lumen of the colon like a tick. They are sometimes covered by unimpaired

epithelium; sometimes the center is excavated, giving an umbilicated appearance. Some of them have ulcerated, giving a follicular ulcer. The muscular coat is sometimes greatly thickened as a result of the muscular work of frequent bowel movement. Sometimes it is atrophied.

Histology: The covering of epithelium on the mucosa is imperfect; where it is present the cells are indifferent in shape. The mucosa is moderately inflamed, partially filled with round .cells and the relations of the glands are abnormal. The glands, which ordinarily lie just on the border line between the mucosa and submucosa, are filled with round cells, and the center may be caseating. If the form is ulcerating the follicular locations represent depressions with follicular walls.

THE APPENDIX.

This has a histology identical with that of the large intestine. It is subject to exactly the same processes, but by reason of the smallness of its lumen, frequently conditions arise which prevent the draining of both pathological and normal products. The intestine is prone to suppurative process, but its mean of exit is never stopped. As a re-

sult of ulceration involving the circumference
a stricture is formed, and contraction of the
inflammatory connective tissue in the submucosa shuts off the lower part of the appendix,
or the appendix may be stopped by a foreign
body; or it may fail to empty itself from muscular atrophy, for it must work against gravity; or it becomes twisted or turned so as to
obliterate the lumen. In the event that a
suppurating process is then going on, the pus
can not drain away, and the organisms are
carried by the lymphatics into the surrounding connective tissue or peritoneum. In the
event that infection has not taken place the
glandular secretions accumulate until the appendix becomes cystic. This sets up a mechanical irritation, which invites infection of
the contained fluids.

SUPPURATIVE APPENDICITIS.

Etiology: Any of the pus germs, e. g.,
bacillus coli communis, streptococcus, staphylococcus, may be the direct agents; foreign
bodies may be contributing agents.

Philosophy of the process: In the more
violent forms, an acute destructive inflammation. Destruction is more violent in the areas
in which the germs are most abundant. In

infection with bacillus coli communis the mucosa is apt to show comparatively evenly black and sloughing.

In staphylococcus infection there is not infrequently large accumulation of pus in the neighborhood of the appendix.

In streptococcus infection there is more apt to be diffuse peritonitis without large accumulation of pus.

Anatomy: The mucosa is dark red or black, sloughing away in places. The entire wall is swollen. When the appendix is split longitudinally the mucosa rolls out and the concavity becomes the convexity. The odor of gangrene is often apparent.

Histology: There is loss of epithelial covering; the mucosa and submucosa are markedly filled with round cells, with islands of blood here and there. Patches of necrosis are present. The muscular bands are separated by inflammatory cells. The adventitia is acutely and violently inflamed.

In cases of recurring appendicitis there is generally stricture formation at the proximal end causing cyst formation. At the stricture, we find an absence of epithelial covering, or else a few scattered indifferent epithelial cells; underneath this is a mass of laminated ma-

tured fibrous tissue, running around the lumen of the tube and parallel with the mucous surface. If this is at the distal end of the tube, there is no cystic accumulation, of course.

The media of the intestine is subject to waxy degeneration.

The tumors to which the intestines are subject are: Lipoma; fibroma; myoma; lymphangioma; angioma; papilloma; simple adenoma; sarcoma; lympho-sarcoma; epithelioma (near the anus); alveolar carcinoma; columnar carcinoma. The tendency of carcinoma in this locality is to become colloid, because the cells from which it begins are mucus-forming cells, or else they readily become mucus-forming cells.

There are certain adventitious diseases, aside from these already spoken of, that affect the intestine.

Invagination is where a slip of intestine from above glides into a slip from below. The condition is more or less physiological; but if it interferes with nutrition, and if muscular effort on the part of the longitudinal fibers does not reduce it, we have sloughing, necrosis, gangrene, intussusception.

Kinking, twisting, turning, incarceration, **either in an inclosed hole, as that into the**

scrotum in hernia, or else behind a band of adhesion, produces pathological processes on the same principle of nutrition "nil."

PERITONEUM.

This has the same histology as the pleura and the pericardium. It is of greater pathological interest, because it is larger, more loose, and between its folds it has a richness in lymphatics and blood vessels that the pleura has not. It is subject to all the infections. By reason of the number of its vessels, and the looseness of the tissue which surrounds them, it is a favorite seat of the noninflammatory transudations from loss of relation (1) between the forces of gravity and heart pressure and (2) between the blood plasma and the connective tissue of the wall.

It has the same varieties of inflammation as the pleura.

Cellular: Dry peritonitis: Productive inflammation with presence of, though not prominence of, exudation.

Exudative.
$$\begin{cases} \text{Serum.} \\ \text{Blood.} \\ \text{Pus.} \\ \text{Adhesions.} \end{cases}$$

The infective granulomata are found in the peritoneum frequently.

Tuberculosis: The process shows beautifully as small pearly nodules with radiating lymphatics.

Histology: Along the course of the small arteries, and the lymphatics, are little nodules, which start as end or periarteritis. The masses are composed of proliferating endothelial cells. If the process is slower, giant cell systems are formed. The histology is the same as tubercle elsewhere.

Carcinoma, adenoma, cystadenoma, papillary cystadenoma, sarcoma, are perhaps the most frequent varieties of tumors of the peritoneum. They are usually secondary. The carcinoma is colloid.

LIVER.

POINTS IN HISTOLOGY.

The liver has both duct and ductless gland functions. To the former system belongs the bile apparatus; to the latter the arrangement of the epithelium into cords radiating from the center to the periphery of the lobule. The liver springs as a bud of the intestinal tract, and in consequence its earliest arrangement is that of a racemose gland. Soon, however, the perivascular arrangement into cords overshadows everything else. The portal branches, known as the peripheral veins, divide into the capillaries of the lobule, and these in turn empty into the central vein; the branches from the portal vein mingle with the branches of the hepatic artery in the lobule. The lobule is the liver unit; for convenience we arbitrarily divide it into three zones, the central zone, the middle zone, and the peripheral zone.

The capsule of the liver is dense and closely adherent.

ACUTE PARENCHYMATOUS HEPATITIS.

Synonym: Cloudy swelling.

Etiology: It is due to poisons brought to the liver by the blood vessels; organic poisons, e. g., those of typhoid fever, scarlet fever, pernicious anæmia, the infectious fevers, septicæmia, pyæmia, etc.; the inorganic poisons, e. g., iodoform, iodol, phosphorus, arsenic.

Philosophy of the process: The process is an inflammatory degeneration, the irritation being just within the limits for the epithelial cell and without the limits for the connective tissue cell. The irritation ending, the albuminous granules in some of the cells go into solution, in others they undergo fatty degeneration, in others the cells undergo some form of death, followed by absorption.

Anatomy: The liver is enlarged and pale; capsule tense; the central vein shows more distinctly than normal.

Histology: The liver cells are swollen, granular, and rounded. The cells stain poorly. The capillary spaces are markedly diminished in size. In this stage the granules are soluble in acetic acid. Later the nucleus begins to lose its staining capacity, and still later all cell outlines are lost.

Sequelæ: Fatty degeneration.

ACUTE DIFFUSE HEPATITIS.

Etiology: An irritation a shade more violent than the preceding, affecting the connective tissues as well as the parenchyma; organic poisons, e. g., severer cases of smallpox, scarlet fever, diphtheria, typhoid.

Philosophy of the process: Cloudy swelling of the highly differentiated parenchyma, non-exudative, productive inflammation of the lowly differentiated tissues. This condition is closely akin to, and merges imperceptibly into, hypertrophic cirrhosis, but differ radically from atrophic cirrhosis. Under the microscope it differs only in degree from miliary abscess. In diffuse hepatitis the fountain of the poison is located outside the liver; in abscess it is in situ. The process is the same in character up to the point where in abscess breaking down becomes prominent.

Anatomy: The liver is enlarged, pale. The capsule is tense. More than the usual amount of blood is found in the portal spaces; there are points of red or gelatinous appearance in the portal space. If these places are small, the liver cannot be told from cloudy swelling; if large, from miliary abscess.

Histology: There is the cloudy swelling of the epithelial cells perviously described. In the connective tissues are islands of round cells; these patches are sometimes rounded and sometimes in bands extending along the capillary walls.

ABSCESS.

The liver is a filter for the portal area. This area is in direct · contact with the external world. It is moist and warm; therefore it is always infected. Contrary to the arrangement of the skin and bronchial tube lining. there is no protection against absorption, but there is rather arrangement for absorption. A very small percentage of the poisonous chemicals absorbed into the portal veins reach the hepatic vein. This is probably true also of the germs that secure entrance.

The abscesses of the liver are of two kinds: (1) multiple and (2) single. The difference between them lies more in the infecting material than in anything else, as the channel of infection is the same in both varieties.

MULTIPLE ABSCESS.

Synonyms: Pyæmic abscess; bacterial necrosis; infection.

Etiology: Some of the forms of pus germs.

Under this head we include infections with organisms that are not usually pyogenic, e. g., the typhoid and diphtheria bacilli.

Philosophy of the process: The liver is much less frequently the seat of abscess in pyæmia than are the other organs, because the portal blood has already passed through one set of capillaries and the hepatic arteries are relatively small in size. Most frequently the source of infection is in the gastro-intestinal tract. Those abscesses due to pus germs give the phenomenon of abscess formation elsewhere, except for the general rule that all dead tissue in the liver becomes bile stained. Those abscesses due to other germs, e. g., the typhoid bacillus, give areas of necrosis with a limited amount of leucocytic reaction.

Anatomy: The liver is pale and in a state of cloudy swelling. On cut section, multiple abscesses, ranging from a pin point to bean size; they may be bile stained (green or yellow), or red and gelatinous. Pus may flow. They may be cheesy or calcareous. If they make cavities, these cavities are wall-less. When the organism is the bacillus typhosus, pus is unusual.

Histology: The histology is the same as

that of ordinary abscess. In the beginning
the arrangement is, an infected thrombus in
the center; around this degenerating liver
cells and leucocytes; some free nuclei; much
tissue detritus; around this. granular epithelium; breaking down and massing of leucocytes; further out leucocytic massing, dilated
congested vessels, liver epithelium. shows
cloudy swelling.

SOLITARY ABSCESS.

Synonyms: Tropical abscess; amœbic abscess.

Etiology: Infection with amœba coli in
the majority of instances. In these cases
there is oftentimes a primary colonic infection.

Philosophy of the process: The cause of
this process is destructive to the liver cells
and at the same time is very slightly irritating
to other tissues. Special irritation.

Anatomy: The abscess is usually single.
It may project above the surface; peritoneal
adhesions bind it to the diaphragm, or to any
of the neighboring viscera. The cavity sometimes opens through the diaphragm into the
pleura or into a bronchial tube. It may open
into the stomach, or intestine, or abdominal

wall, or into the peritoneum. The cavity has a ragged, uneven wall. The pus is reddish, somewhat like prune-juice.

Histology: There is little connective tissue in the abscess wall.

CHRONIC INFLAMMATIONS.

We will study first that interstitial lesion in the liver which is most marked and presents the most salient points.

ATROPHIC CIRRHOSIS.

Synonyms: Common cirrhosis; alcoholic cirrhosis; sclerosis of the liver; gin drinker's liver; granular liver; hob-nail liver.

Etiology: A mild irritation long continued, an irritant affecting the connective tissues only, and borne to the liver, in greatest part, by the portal veins. Such an irritation is produced by alcohol or ether, taken into the gastro-intestinal tract, or manufactured by fermentation processes therein.

Philosophy of the process: The poison is carried to the liver by the portal vein. In consequence it is in the vicinity of the portal structures—the interlobular spaces—that the lesion first manifests itself. It is a blood-vessel-wall disease, and all the effects, and therefore all the symptoms, are due, not to

the inflammatory process, for the structures inflamed are of minor importance, but to the thickening of the vascular walls and to the secondary contraction that characterizes all inflammatory connective tissue.

Associated with cirrhosis is always marked fatty change, for two reasons. In the first place, there cannot be a proper liver work through thick-walled capillaries; in the second place, the alcoholics, in whom cirrhosis is found, are prone to obesity.

Anatomy: The liver is diminished in size. No other affection, except acute yellow atrophy, gives a small liver. The capsule is thickened and firmly adherent. To the touch the liver is hard. The scarring is the most striking feature. The surface is covered in whole or in part by small elevations about the size of a hob-nail, or shoe nail head. Some of the eminences may be of large size. The fissures that mark the eminences are hard and paler. On cut section the liver is usually yellow. It may be pale and perceptibly fatty. The capsule can be seen sending trabeculæ into the substance. The section cuts and feels firm. The intertrabecular tissue is softer; the trabeculæ are firm, grayish.

Histology: With the low power it will be easily seen that the portal trabeculæ are markedly increased in size. The inner layers will be old; the layers next the lobules will be more nucleated; at the periphery of the lobule it will be apparent that the connective tissue is "shaving off" the epithelial cells. Some of the lobules will be nothing but small islands.

With the high power the increase in connective tissue at the edge of the trabeculæ will be evident. In some foci this tissue will be round cell tissue. The bulk of it will be fibrillated connective tissue, but with a considerable number of spindle nuclei. In its meshes are ribbons of epithelial cells, usually compressed. These cells resist degenerations longer than the cells of the remainder of the lobule; they are recognizable as liver epithelium until compression is very advanced. Beyond this zone there is proliferation of the connective tissue between the liver cells. While the process is more marked in the periphery of the lobule, it can in some lobules be seen to reach to the center; but near the center the cells are round or spindles or young fibers. The epithelial cells are usually very fatty. In some the fat is in granules, but usually it is

in globules. Signet ring cells are the rule. The new development of bile capillaries among the liver cells is not prominent. In fact the epithelium is undergoing very little inflammatory reaction. In the bands of the connective tissue there are found considerable numbers of bile capillaries, and occasionally these are seen extending into the liver cell areas; but as a general thing the liver cells are fatty and nothing more.

Effects: Venous congestion effects in the abdominal area, e. g., ascites, hæmorrhage into the stomach and intestines, hæmorrhoids; loss of liver function, deficient urea.

Tendency: It is progressive; usually progressive by invasion by inflammatory connective tissue, but always progressive by contraction of inflammatory connective tissue.

HYPERTROPHIC CIRRHOSIS.

Synonyms: Biliary cirrhosis; monolobular cirrhosis.

Etiology: A mild irritation long continued. The irritant affects both the connective tissue and the epithelial cell.

Philosophy of the process: We have a productive inflammation in both the parenchyma of the organ and in its interstitial tissue. The

effects are spread throughout the lobule much more evenly. Tying the bile duct in lower animals has produced this form of cirrhosis. The liver epithelium in its embryonal form was a columnar epithelium lining a duct; when it is irritated, as in this affection, it has a tendency to arrange itself in tubular form and assume columnar shape. As the epithelium is affected liver function is rapidly interfered with, and death comes before time is had for atrophic changes.

Anatomy: The liver is greatly enlarged at times. The capsule is but little thickened. The surface is irregular, but the elevations are very uniform in size. The liver "cuts" tough; cut section looks granular and bile stained.

Histology: The round and spindle cells are found throughout the lobule, although not as abundant in the center as at the periphery. There is not the same massing of large quantities of connective tissue as seen in the atrophic form. Some of the liver cells are swollen and granular; some are dividing. In the connective tissue there is an unusually large number of bile capillaries; at the margins of the connective tissue, the liver cells, cubical in shape, are arranging themselves as double columns—bile capillaries.

CHRONIC VENOUS CONGESTION.

Synonyms: Nutmeg liver; liver of heart disease; cyanotic atrophy.

Etiology: This form of chronic interstitial hepatitis is due to long continued venous stasis from obstruction to the return of blood to the heart; e. g., valvular lesions of the heart, long continued; pleurisy with effusion; tumors of the lung; emphysema.

Philosophy of the process: The damming of blood causes stasis in the central vein of lobule, and thence in the capillaries running into it. The vessels then are chronically dilated and the liver effects are due to (1) pressure, (2) nutrition minus, (3) prolonged contact with the leucomaines representing tissue waste. Here, as well as in all venous congestions, there is a minus condition of the highly differentiated parenchyma, and a plus condition of the lowly differentiated connective tissue.

Anatomy: Capsule tense, thin. On cut section the liver lobule shows very plainly. The central zone is dark red; the middle and outer zone is pale and fatty. Later we find irregular patches of connective tissue, and the contraction effects of such bands.

Histology: The central veins and the

radiating capillaries are distended. The enclosed cells are shrunken and pigmented. This inner zone is called the zone of nutmeg changes. Later there is an overgrowth of connective tissue, attended by further compression of the liver cells. The middle and outer zones are fatty.

TUBERCULOSIS OF THE LIVER.

Etiology: Tubercle bacillus.

Philosophy of the process: Tuberculosis presents no peculiarities here. It very frequently makes giant cells. It is stained green or yellow from bile while still small.

Anatomy: The liver may show cloudy swelling; scattered throughout, but more abundant near the capsule and in the portal spaces, are small nodules, gray at first, later green.

Histology: In or near the center is a giant cell with multiple nuclei; from some portion of its periphery, trabeculæ run out among the surrounding cells. Outside this is a massing of round cells with some reticulum. At the margin these connective tissue cells and leucocytes can be seen growing among the liver cells, while liver cells are showing evidence of degeneration. The tubercular

nodules are found toward the periphery of the liver lobule.

SYPHILIS.

Syphilis of the liver begins as a diffuse sclerosis with marked increase in the connective tissue—the portal areas. There are the usual contraction effects in the parenchyma. It spends much of its force on blood vessels, so that there is abundant making of capillary loops. This same irritation of vessel walls causes thickening of the vessel wall as it grows older, and finally an obliteration by endarteritis obliterans. With this the stage of gumma is reached.

GUMMATA.

Anatomy: The tumor may reach considerable size. It may be multiple, but it frequently is single. It is most frequently on the surface, and often near the suspensory ligament. Early it is rose gray; later it is green. It has a capsule, which capsule is intimately connected with the surrounding tissue. This is always marked in syphilitic capsules. The contents are apt to be grumous.

DEGENERATIONS OF THE LIVER.

CLOUDY SWELLING.

Treated under acute parenchymatous inflammation.

FATTY DEGENERATION.

Etiology: It is found as a later stage of cloudy swelling, and therefore due to the same causes; organic poisons—toxins of continued fevers, Addison's disease, pernicious anæmia, phthisis, cancer, etc.; inorganic poisons—phosporus, arsenic, iodoform, antimony, alcohol, ether.

Philosophy of the process: It is a degeneration, conforming to the general laws of fatty degeneration. The liver is a favorite seat because of its position with relation to the intestines, and also because the liver is the great toxin destroyer of the body. It represents faulty internal oxidation.

Anatomy: The liver is somewhat decreased in size, in weight and in specific gravity. On section it is pale.

Histology: **The liver cells are shrunken,**

angular, and contain granules of fat. These dissolve in ether, stain black with osmic acid. In specimens prepared in the ordinary way, the areas of former fat shows as small clear points, or vesicles.

Note.—To get the ether and osmic reactions the specimens must be taken fresh and treated with these agents as the first step in handling.

FATTY INFILTRATION.

Far the more frequent of the fatty processes. It is always pathological, but not necessarily symptomatically so, nor even usually symptomically so.

Synonyms: Lipomatosis; adiposis.

Etiology: Alcohol; fatty or starchy diet; maltose; sugars.

Philosophy of the process: It is due to external error; that is to say, the liver protoplasm itself is not changed into fat. Fatty liver, presenting all the characteristics of fatty infiltration, is found in many diseases accompanied by great emaciation. It is regularly found when there is a lack of relation between food taken and exercise. This is true not only of carbonaceous foods, but also of nitrogenous diet.

Anatomy: The liver is large, firm. It pits on pressure and these pits remain. It is increased in weight and decreased in specific gravity. The organ is pale yellow in color. It is greasy, and scrapings will float as grease on the surface of the water.

Histology: In specimens prepared in alcohol, etc., the liver lobule shows as a meshwork enclosing holes of various sizes, up to somewhat larger than a liver cell. Close examination shows the liver protoplasm pushed as a delicate ring around this clear zone; at one point the nucleus is seen as a projecting mass. In the later stages the lobule is about evenly affected. Frequently the process begins in the external third of the liver lobule, so this is called the zone of fatty infiltration. This distribution is by no means constant.

Effects: Slight; life processes are but little interfered with. A certain degree of fatty infiltration is entirely physiological.

WAXY LIVER.

Synonyms: Waxlike liver; amyloid, lardaceous, bacony liver.

Etiology: Long continued suppuration; phthisis, empyema, leucocythæmia, dysentery, **syphilis.**

Philosophy of the process: An infiltration of the connective tissue, and especially of the capillary wall, with a modified albumin. The only effects on the liver cells are (1) nutrition effects from the relatively impermeable vessel wall, and (2) pressure effects.

Anatomy: The liver is very large—sometimes twice its normal size. It is heavy and increased in specific gravity. The contour is rounded. The capsule thin and tense. It pits on pressure, but the pits are soon lost. Cut surface is pale, shiny, waxlike, or dull pink. The lobules are indistinct. Thin sections with a double-bladed knife show waxy areas. These stain brown with iodine.

Histology: The capillary walls are widely distended with a homogeneous substance; no tissue except the nuclei show in the areas, but the nuclei show very distinctly. The liver cells may be compressed into apparent solid cords. The process begins in the capillaries of the middle third of the lobule; this is, therefore, called the zone of waxy infiltration.

ACUTE YELLOW ATROPHY.

Synonyms: Icterus gravus.

Etiology: Not known; found most frequently in young pregnant women.

Philosophy of the process. There is a substance which is violently toxic to the liver epithelium, and is nonirritating to the connective tissue.

Anatomy: The liver is markedly decreased in size, weighing about thirty-five ounces. Its capsule is wrinkled. It "cuts" tough, and cut section is ochre yellow with islands of deep bile staining.

Histology: The network of connective tissue stands out very plainly. But slight evidence of proliferation is found in this. The liver cells are indistinct in outline, most of them simply being masses of granular debris. The cells and their nuclei stain very poorly; crystals of leucin and tyrosin can sometimes be found.

TUMORS OF THE LIVER.

The liver is the seat of multiple (1) congenital cysts, (2) retention cysts, (3) ecchinococcus cysts. It is a favorite site of both angioma telangiectoides and angioma cavernosa.

SARCOMATA.

When primary anywhere in the intestinal tract, they are very apt to give secondary growths in the liver. These are frequently

melanotic. The tumors are generally nodular, multiple, soft, not umbilicated, and cut section shows islands of hæmorrhages.

CARCINOMATA.

This is a frequent secondary tumor in the liver. It may be carried from almost any locality by lymphatics, by blood vessels, and along bile channels. The more frequent point of origin is the stomach, lower end of œsophagus, and upper end of the duodenum. The nodules are usually large, umbilicated. Around the nodules, and sometimes in areas some distance removed from the nodules, the liver is honeycombed; that is, the liver cells are broken down, as in acute yellow atrophy, and the connective tissue stands out more prominently. The carcinoma tends to assume the same arrangement of epithelium as in the areas from which it sprung.

ADENOMATA.

Are sometimes found in the lower animals; coccidium oviforme produces a typical adenoma.

Angiomata find here one of their most frequent sites.

THE KIDNEY.

The kidney is a tubular gland in which the tube begins at the Malpighian corpuscle and ends at the apex of the pyramid. In the cortex are found all the convoluted tubules and some of the straight tubules. In the medulla are found most of the straight tubules. The blood supply of the kidney is remarkably rich. The space between the tubules is filled with blood vessels and a small amount of connective tissue. The tubes are lined by epithelial cells. The kidneys are derived from the Wolffian bodies, and these in turn from the mesoblast. The markings are due to the alternating blood vessels and uriniferous tubules.

The lesions of the kidney are due to inflammations, degenerations, tumors and developmental errors.

Inflammations.

Acute.

(1) Cloudy swelling.

Synonyms: Acute parenchymatous, nephri-

tis, acute parenchymatous degeneration, acute Bright's disease, molecular degeneration.

Etiology: Toxæmias, especially those in which the poison is eliminated by the kidney. All acute febrile conditions, severe in type, e. g., septicæmia, scarlet fever, measles, small-pox, yellow fever; inorganic poisons, e. g., phosphorus, arsenic, carbolic acid, iodoform, chloroform and ether.

Philosophy of the process: The same as cloudy swelling elsewehere. It is an inflammatory degeneration and may return to normal or progress to fatty degeneration or necrosis, resulting in granular debris. It is to be borne in mind that it is the channel by which the poison leaves a body that is most affected by it, for its excretion means a special irritability on the part of that cell toward that particular poison. This physiological irritability increased gives pathological irritability.

Anatomy: The kidney is enlarged and pale. Its capsule strips off easily; the stellate veins show distinctly. On cut section the thickening is seen to be in the cortex. The markings show plainly; the Malpighian corpuscles, being filled with blood, are accentuated.

The medulla is not markedly affected.

Histology: The tubes, especially the convoluted tubes, are widely dilated. The epithelium is so swollen as to obliterate the lumen in many tubules—to decrease it in all. The outline of the individual cell cannot be made out. The nucleus stains well with a nuclear stain, such as hæmatoxylon. Casts are seen in many of the tubes. The connective tissue is unaffected.

Vessels: The Malpighian tuft fills the capsule. In some cases, merging into the next form, there is marked dilation of the vessels and exudation of red cells into the connective tissue and into the surrounding tubes.

Sequelæ: This form of nephritis gives scanty urine, containing albumin, casts and epithelial cells. It never proceeds to chronic inflammations.

ACUTE DIFFUSE NEPHRITIS.

Synonyms: Acute exudative nephritis; acute Bright's disease; acute desquamative nephritis.

Etiology: Toxæmias a shade more violent than those of cloudy swelling, e. g., scarlet fever, diphtheria, etc.; turpentine, etc.

Philosophy of the process; The principle involved is that of general irritability. As a

rule the more highly specialized chemically-functioning epithelium is breaking down—destructive inflammation—whilst the more lowly differentiated connective tissue is in a state of productive inflammation. Being a productive inflammation, it is much more liable to produce chronic disorder than is parenchymatous nephritis.

Anatomy: Capsule tense, peels off easily, kidney swollen, redder than in acute parenchymatous; moist. Red patches are seen here and there. Glomeruli distinct, markings distinct. Stellate veins stand out prominently; cortex thickened; markings distinct; show glomeruli and islands of hæmorrhage, as pinkish points. Mucous membrane of the pelvis injected. It is difficult with the naked eye to distinguish this kidney from its predecessor, because they merge imperceptibly into each other.

Histology: (a) Epithelium: The epithelium is in about the same condition as in parenchymatous nephritis, swollen, granular, filling the tube, falling away from the basement membrane. In the tubes are casts, hyalin, granular, epithelial and blood.

Vessels and connective tissue: A Malpighian tuft fills the capsule, there may be an in-

crease in the tuft cells. Islands of extravasated blood can be seen sometimes among the capillaries of the tuft. The capsule is thickened by round cell proliferation, and this extends into the adjoining connective tissue.

(b) Interlobular vessels: In formalin prepared specimens the arteries are dilated; islands of extravasated blood are found in the connective tissue and in the tubes. The walls and other connective tissue are thickened by round cells, leucocytes and connective tissue cells. The exuded plasma may be coagulated in the connective tissue, in which event the tissues give the homogeneous appearance of amyloid. The staining reactions differentiate them.

Variations: If the process is violent there is a large exudatoin of red cells and the process is called hæmorrhagic nephritis.

In scarlet fever the poison spends its greatest force on the glomerulus and the disease is known as glomerular nephritis. The other tissues are involved as in diffuse nephritis. The maximum of intensity is found in the glomerulus. This variety is very prone to eventuate in chronic interstitial nephritis.

SUPPURATIVE NEPHRITIS.

Two forms.   Pyæmic and pyelonephritic.

PYÆMIC KIDNEY.

Synonyms: Multiple abscess of the kidney; embolic abscess; miliary abscess.

Etiology: Infection with some of the organisms that produce pus, or that can produce pus in this locality, either as usually existing or as modified by circumstances. These include streptococcus, staphylococcus, pneumococcus, bacillus coli communis, bacillus typhosus.

Philosophy of the process: The route of infection is the blood current. The process is the destructive inflammation usual in abscess formation. In the area more remote, where the poison is dilute, we may have productive inflammation or cloudy swelling. The kidney is a frequent site because of its large blood supply, its double set of capillaries, and the tortuosity of the capillaries in the tuft. Not all abscesses are symptomatic, nor necessarily fatal.

Anatomy: The kidney is usually enlarged, pale and moist. The capsule strips easily. On cut section there is a varying pallor, interspread with multiple millet seed foci, red or white or yellow in color, and purulent. These are seldom larger than 2 mm. across. While they are sometimes round, they have a tendency to be elongated. They are located in the cortex. Some of these foci are recognizable as abscesses filled with pus.

Histology: The foci show a central mass of pus corpuscles and around this a typical inflammation, some gradually merging into the surrounding tissue. In these areas the fixed elements, epithelium, connective tissue, etc., are degenerating, granular, fragmenting nuclei, etc. The areas of usual involvement are the tufts and the intertubular vessels. The tubules away from the zone of pus show pus casts and organisms. The cortical tubes show cloudy swelling.

SUPPURATIVE PYELONEPHRITIS.

Synonyms: Surgical kidney; pyelonephrosis.

Etiology: Pus germs traveling from the urethra, bladder or ureter to the pelvis of the kidney, thence along the lymph spaces be-

tween the uriniferous tubules to medulla, later to the cortex, rarely to the perinephritic tissue.

Philosophy of the process: This is much the more frequent and the more important form of nephritis. The kidney may be converted into multilocular cysts, or by liquefaction of the capsule, extension externally may be produced. Pus germs can only travel through the capsule by liquefaction. The putrefaction in the urine causes deposits in the pelvis or ureter, and these calculi cause a persistence of the infection which otherwise the leucocytes might overcome.

Anatomy: The kidney is large, red, moist, friable. It may be cystic. The capsule usually strips off easily. On cut section striæ and foci of abscess formation can be seen in the medulla extending sometimes to the cortex. The pelvis is dilated, with thick walls. The cavity is filled with pus. Calculi are not infrequent. The ureters are widely dilated, and with irregularly thickened walls.

Histology: That of abscess formation: granulation tissue, and destruction of local tissues. Bands of extension can be seen between the collecting tubes of the medullary pyramids.

Chronic inflammation of the kidneys. We will study first the extreme type.

CHRONIC INTERSTITIAL NEPHRITIS.

Synonyms: Granular contracted kidney; cirrhosis of the kidney: sclerosis; small red kidney; gouty kidney; chronic indurative nephritis; arterio sclerotic kidney.

Etiology: A mild irritation long continued, borne to the kidney by the vessels, and affecting the vessel wall and the perivascular connective tissue; chronic alcoholism, gout.

Philosophy of the process: The process is the same as in cirrhosis of various other organs, e. g., liver, brain, cord. It is due to mild irritation from leucomaines or substances similar in the scale of toxicity. To the same class belong the lesions of age. In old age there is frequently more obliterating endarteritis. Like cirrhosis elsewhere, the process is uneven in wedge-shaped masses in the kidney, in irregular bands in the liver, in disseminated plaques in multiple sclerosis of the cord or brain. The epithelium in the patches of sclerosis is compressed and angular and disappears from many tubules so as to show as an obliterated tube, but when examined microscopically is is found as much the

healthiest epithelium in the kidney. Death in all cases ensues from some form of terminal infection, giving cloudy swelling of the epithelium between the tubes. The affection is of the vessel wall, and in consequence kidney functions are imperfectly performed. For this same reason the irritant that causes cloudy swelling of the epithelium of the normal tubes does not affect that of the compressed tube.

Secondary atrophy of tubules after affections of glomeruli.

Anatomy: The kidney is very small, weighing from one and a half to three ounces. The capsule is thick and laminated. The surface is very granular, leathery in appearance. In the aged this roughing is more irregular. When the capsule is torn off, it may split in layers, leaving a smooth surface behind, or else it tears off with difficulty, bringing with it pieces of kidney. On cut section multiple cortical cysts are seen, varying in size from a millet seed to a marble. The cyst walls are smooth. The contents are either clear water or colloid. The kidney "cuts" tough. The cortex is markedly thinned. The striations are obscured or not apparent. The arteries **have thick, rigid walls.**

Histology: There wedge-shaped masses of fibrillated connective tissue, denser and less nucleated in the center than at the periphery. There are pin point holes, remnants of kidney tubes; other tubes that are larger contain several cells, showing multiple nuclei that are distinct, but in which the cell outlines cannot be differentiated. Others, and these comprise the bulk of the tubules, show a ring of epithelial cells staining distinctly. Some of the glomeruli are converted into a solid mass of connective tissue, and others show only a capsular thickening. The vessels in these central areas show as irregular clefts whose walls merge intimately into the surrounding connective tissue. At the periphery of these wedges there are embryonal cells, round and spindle. These areas, and especially the glomeruli, are frequently infiltrated with coagulated plasma, giving the appearance of amyloid; this to be differentiated by special staining. Between these wedges the tubules are widely dilated, and the epithelium is in a state of cloudy swelling. In this area we not infrequently find foci of acute round cell infiltration. Here the terminal infection has been with a pus germ.

Variations.

The large white kidney of chronic inflammation.

It is difficult to write clearly of this symposium of lesions, because there is no clear-cut line by which it can be subdivided, and it thus stretches by easy gradations from acute nephritis with increase in bulk, to the maturing lesions of chronic nephritis with a small kidney.

Synonyms: Fatty kidney; chronic parenchymatous nephritis; subacute Bright's disease; large mottled kidney.

Etiology: Mild irritations, long continued, in which the epithelium is pathologically irritated. It may follow acute diffuse forms or glomerular nephritis. Generally it is found existent without any history of a beginning.

Philosophy: Beginning as a diffuse nephritis, caused by an irritant that is pathological to kidney epithelium, it cannot, and does not, last long enough for the connective tissue to mature and develop either pressure effects or sufficient density to wholly prevent interchange of nutrition elements. Much of its pathology is dependent upon the principle that a breaking down of highly differentiated elements is followed by an overgrowth of lowly differentiated connective tissue.

Anatomy: Early stages—Kidney large, sometimes double the normal size. It is smooth; capsule slightly thickened and moderately adherent. The surface is pale and mottled with distinct stellate veins. Cut surface shows a thickened, pale, yellowish or reddish yellow cortex, mottled with islands of hæmorrhage.

Late stages—The kidney is normal in size or mildly decreased. The capsule thickened and moderately adherent. The surface is mottled and irregular. There are depressions and elevations, but the granular appearance is nothing like so typical as in the variety called chronic interstitial nephritis. The kidney cuts tough; a few cortical cysts are found. The cortex is thinned; the markings indistinct.

Histology: *a* Epithelium: The epithelium is in a state of cloudy swelling, or loose in the tubules. In many of the tubes the epithelium is entirely gone. Casts of all kinds are found in the tubes.

Vessels and connective tissue: In the glomeruli, and in the vessels making up the tube walls, there is an increase of connective tissue in spindles and fibers. It differs from the other variety, in that there is not the

same extensive blocking of everything by connective tissue and in the greater abundance of young connective tissue elements.

TUBERCULOSIS OF THE KIDNEY.

Two kinds: Miliary and tubercular pyelonephritis.

MILIARY TUBERCULOSIS.

Route of infection: Blood vessels.

Philosophy of the process: That of miliary tubercle elsewhere. In this form of kidney tuberculosis there is a general miliary tuberculosis, and in consequence the kidney shows cloudy swelling. Again, the patient does not long survive; hence the lesions are usually found in the round cell stage.

Anatomy: The kidney may be slightly increased in size and pale. Underneath the capsule and generally in the cortex or multiple millet seed, gray, gelatinous or yellow tubercles.

Histology: The histology is that of a small tubercle in its round cell stage. Exceptionally there are giant cell systems. The tubercles are found along the interlobular arteries.

TUBERCULAR PYELONEPHRITIS.

Route of infection: Up the lymphatics of the lower urinary apparatus.

Philosophy: Attention is directed to the similarity in tuberculosis to infection with pus microbes. In this form of tuberculosis we find even distribution of the lesions rather than the nodular arrangement of the miliary tubercle. A similar appearance is seen in some cases of tubercular bronchitis. It is due to the attending pus infection. The nodules are joined together by masses of streptococcus, staphylococcus, or other germ inflammation. They then belong in the same category as phthisis, as distinguished from lung tuberculosis.

Anatomy: Both kidneys are usually affected. The ureters are usually widely dilated and have thick walls. The pelvis of the kidney is dilated. We are apt to find pus in the pelvis. The kidney may be converted into one or multiple cysts. The pelvic mucosa is rather evenly thickened and whitish, or yellowish and dirty There are tubercular nodules, most prominent in the medulla, but found also in the cortex; calculi are found.

Histology: We find tubercular nodules in the pyramids between the tubules. There are giant cell systems more frequently than in miliary tubercle. The mucosa of the pelvis is covered by lime deposits. Underneath

this are tubercular nodules and surrounding these diffuse, round cell infiltration. The epithelial covering cannot be demonstrated.

Syphilis: The syphilitic granuloma shows a marked tendency to develop into gummata.

WAXY KIDNEY.

Synonyms: Amyloid; lardaceous.

Etiology: Prolonged suppuration; phthisis with cavities; empyema; syphilis; leucocythæmia; Addison's disease.

Philosophy of the process: As elsewhere, it is an infiltration of the vessel walls with lardacein, which albumin coagulates there. If the albumin goes through into the tube and remains in solution, it reacts as albumin in the urine; that which coagulates in the tube gives a cast, that which coagulates in the tissue gives the lesion now described.

Anatomy: The kidney is very much enlarged, up to twice its normal size. The capsule strips easily, leaving a smooth, brownish yellow surface, mottled with lighter areas. On section the cortex is thickened, and the glomeruli stand out as glistening masses. Thin sections cut with a Valentine knife show intertubular bands and glomeruli of translucent material. This, stained with

iodine, shows brown. The papillæ are very pale. The boundary zone is deeper in color.

Histology: Epithelium unaffected.

Vessels and connective tissue: In the tufts in which the process is just beginning one or two of the capillary loops show as thick homogeneous bands, the nuclei showing distinctly. In others the tuft is a mass of homogeneous material, showing no structure but the nuclei. The capsule is infiltrated. The epithelium of the tubes rests on a thickened basement membrane. This epithelium is granular and falls away. The change is very marked in the arteriæ rectæ near the tip of the pyramid. Staining reaction with iodine and sulphuric acid; with methylanilin violet and oxalic acid.

Pyonephrosis. In this condition there is suppuration of the pelvis with dilatation.

Hydronephrosis. This is a dilatation of the pelvis with urine.

Cystic Kidney. This is a congenital affection in which the kidney (usually both) is converted into a mass of cysts of comparatively uniform size. No stoppage of the ureter is discoverable. It is sometimes difficult to diagnose any kidney stroma with the

unaided eye. Microscopically we find the septa composed of kidney stroma.

Cysts of the kidney and hydronephrosis are due to obstruction somewhere between the glomerulus and the glans penis. The more frequent causes are stricture of the urethra, calculus, enlarged prostate, cystitis, malformations of the bladder, pelvic tumors, stricture of the ureter, organic, or due to bending or kinking, tumors, chronic interstitial nephritis, suppuration of the pelvis. The kidney may be converted into one large somewhat kidney shaped cyst, or into any number of smaller cysts.

Movable kidney is frequently movable behind the peritoneum. A floating kidney has grown into the peritoneum, gaining a mesentery.

Tumors: The kidney is the seat of malignant growths much more frequently than it is of nonmalignant growths. It can be assumed that any tumor of appreciable size is malignant. It is subject to both sarcomata and carcinomata.

GONORRHŒAL URETHRITIS.

Etiology: Gonococcus, not infrequently associated with other pus cocci.

Philosophy of the process: This organism is essentially an epithelial organism. Its toxin absorbs, producing some inflammatory reaction in the lymph channels in which it travels, and also general toxæmia. When strictures result, there is probably secondary infection of the submucosa with other germs. It is prone to wander into the crypts of glands, and there lose its virulency, sometimes to regain it on proper occasion, sometimes never.

Anatomy: The membrane is covered by yellow pus; it is red, moist, swollen. There is some injection of the corpora and of the glans.

Histology: The surface layers of epithelium are irregular in shape, falling away. The deep layers are actively dividing. Along the lymphatics and capillaries of the submucosa, there is mild round cell infiltration.

STRICTURE.

Etiology: Gonorrhœa; trauma.

Philosophy of the process: Maturing inflammatory connective tissue in the submucosa.

Histology: Bands of fibrillated connective tissue encircle the lumen, decreasing it. The

epithelial covering may be normal; it may be thickened with irregular cells; it may be absent.

Epispadias: A malformation in which the urethra opens on the top of the penis, back of the glans.

Hypospadias: A malformation in which the urethra opens under the penis, back of the glans.

SYPHILIS.

The lesions of syphilis are divided into three groups:

1. Primary—chancres, mucous patches.
2. Secondary—the roseola, skin eruption.
3. Tertiary—granulomata, similar to tuberculosis, actinomycosis and sarcoma.

CHANCRE.

1. Primary.

Synonyms: Chancre, mucous patches.

Etiology: A specific organism, not yet determined; the Lustgarten bacillus is not accepted.

Philosophy of the process: It is a granuloma, a productive inflammation, nonexudative in character. Destruction and ulceration is secondary.

 Anatomy: The sore is indurated with a

hard, raised edge. It is "punched out;" is pyramidal in shape with its base at the skin surface.

Histology: The more superficial layers of the corium are proliferating actively. The blood vessels are moderately distended with blood. There is inflammation in the vessel wall.

2. Secondary.

The erythemas—

Philosophy of the process: The lesions are those of toxæmia, and give the same anatomy and histology, varying in degree only, as other toxæmias, such as fish poisoning, measles, scarlet fever.

3. Tertiary.

Philosophy of the process: A granuloma as in tubercle, sarcoma, actinomycosis. The spindle cells have little tendency to mature into fibers. There is a great tendency to some of the forms of death, simple necrosis, formation of fat, caseation. There is less disposition to secondary infection with pus germs than in tuberculosis. There is a greater prominence of arteritis. This in some measure accounts for the prominence of the various forms of death.

DISEASES OF THE BLADDER.

ACUTE CYSTITIS.

Etiology: Due to pus germs, to gonococcus, or to milder irritants. Presents no points of peculiarity marking it from other acute inflammations of mucous structures.

Hypertrophy follows dilatation of the bladder.

CHRONIC CYSTITIS.

Differs in no particular from chronic inflammations in other mucous membranes. In this connection see inflammation of the stomach.

There is the great tendency to irregularity of the mucosa in places resulting in polypoid growths, always the tendency in a mucosa which is bathed in moisture, and is chronically inflamed. The urine is acid until after infection with the micrococcus ureæ takes place, when ammonia is produced. This continues the irritation in two ways. In the first place it is in itself an irritant; in the second place it causes a deposit of triple phosphates. The most frequent cause is infection through the urethra; the second, enlarged prostate.

The bladder is found dilated, sometimes with thin walls, but generally with walls immensely thickened.

All suppurative inflammation back of compressor urethræ drains into the bladder.

TUBERCULOSIS IN THE BLADDER.

May be a result of infection from the kidney. It generally involves the base. Very frequently the seminal vesicles are involved. Early involvement of the epididymis and testicle may ensue. The sequence of involvement may be reversed. The lesion is mixed; the tubercular nodules are imbedded in a mass of diffuse granulation tissue, due to the other germs. Ulceration is early and marked. In this it shows resemblance to tubercular pyelo-nephritis, bronchitis and phthisis pulmonalis.

TESTICLE.

The testicle is subject to malformation, malposition, errors in development of the investing membrane, acute and chronic inflammations and tumors.

·ACUTE INFLAMMATIONS.

Acute orchitis may exist without epididymitis, epididymitis without orchitis, or they may exist conjointly.

Etiology: Gonorrhœa, smallpox, mumps, trauma.

Philosophy of the process: Gonorrhœal inflammation tends to limit itself to the epithelium of the tubule. In consequence there is parenchymatous orchitis and subsidence of the disease without permanent pathology. The orchitis of smallpox and of mumps involves the interstitial tissue, and there is far greater tendency to interstitial overgrowth and consequent atrophy. In trauma there are all grades of injury and all shades of results; abscess formation is due to pus germs and is rather unusual except in severe trauma with infection, and in tuberculosis.

Anatomy: The testicle is enlarged, the tunica tense. On section the parenchyma rolls out of its envelope and the tunic side becomes concave. The vessels of the vaginalis are congested; the membrane œdematous.

Histology: The tube is filled with swollen granular epithelial cells. In some cases the interstitial tissue is filled with round cells also. Blood vessels dilated; much œdema of interstitial tissue.

Sequelæ: Gonorrhœal, usually none. Many cases of mumps, and some cases of

trauma and gonorrhœa are followed by atrophy.

TUBERCULAR TESTICLE.

Route of infection: Generally along the spermatic cord and down the tubes; rarely by way of the vessels.

Anatomy: The testicle is enlarged; the epididymis generally participates in the process; most frequently one testicle is involved. On section, scattered tubercular nodules in varying stages, abscess cavities, cheesy zones, yellow nodes, small gray gelatinous miliary points.

Histology: That of tubercle with a large amount of simple inflammation diffusely scattered.

Sequelæ: The abscesses are liable to perforate both albuginea and vaginalis, and, infecting the scrotum, make a persistent sinus. It is very liable to cause a general tubercular infection.

SYPHILIS.

Origin: The disease may be acquired or inherited. In acquired syphilis gummata and necrosis forms are more prominent. In inherited syphilis diffuse sclerosis and atrophic phenomena predominate.

Anatomy: The scrotum is frequently joined to the testicle by close connective tissue investment. Both albuginea and vaginalis are greatly thickened. Some degree of hydrocele is the rule. The mediastinal bands are thickened; there are usually multiple gummata. These grow by preference from the periphery into the interior. The larger masses are cheesy or purulent; they may open externally.

Histology: Bands of connective tissue, old and fibrillated, enclose tubules. Some of these tubules are of small caliber and free from epithelium. The vessels have thickened walls. The gumma is a mass of round and spindle cell granulation tissue. This is oftentimes a mass of granular debris

TUMORS.

Sarcoma: Generally round and spindle cells, and markedly malignant. Cysto-sarcoma are frequent.

Carcinoma: A great preponderance of medullary carcinoma. This may in part be accounted for by the fact that the testicle is almost a purely epithelial structure. Its connective tissue is normally inconsiderable in **amount.**

Chondroma, fibroma, cysts, retention cysts, dermoid cysts are found.

Hydrocele, or water in the tunica, is frequent. It is of three varieties:

1. Congenital hydrocele, in which the connection between the tunica vaginalis and the peritoneal cavity remains patulous and the cavity fills up with peritoneal fluid.

2. Hydrocele proper, in which the connection is obliterated and there is an exudation cyst in the vaginalis proper. It is situated anterior to the testicle.

3. Hydrocele of the cord, in which an island of the peritoneum remains at some point along the vas deferens. The connection with the peritoneum is obliterated, also that with the tunica vaginalis. It is above the testicle.

Varicocele. Cirsoid aneurism of the spermatic veins. It exists by reason of two factors:

1. Frequent congestion of the testicle.
2. The unsupported condition of the veins.

DISEASES OF THE FEMALE GENITAL ORGANS.

POINTS IN HISTOLOGY AND DEVELOPMENT.

From the uro-genital eminence develops the ovary proper. In the vicinity of this develops the Wolffian body. In the Wolffian body the Wolffian duct and Mueller's duct develop as parallel tubes. The Wolffian body develops into the broad ligaments; the Wolffian ducts develop into Gartner's duct, Rosenmueller's ducts and Kobelt's tubes. Mueller's ducts develop into the vagina, the uterus, the Fallopian tubes. The lower end of the Wolffian ducts and Mueller's ducts empty into the allantois. As this hind gut grows toward the surface, the epiblast begins to dent in. Then the two blind sacs coalesce, septa grow down, making separate openings, and the urethra, vagina and rectum are at hand.

Malformations: By reason of failure of some of these steps, we sometimes have imperforate vagina, vesico-vaginal fistula, recto-

vaginal fistula, vesicocele, rectocele, double vagina, double uterus, single Fallopian tube.

Histology: The vulva, vagina and cervix uteri are musculo-fibrous tubes, covered by squamous epithelium. The vulva has race-mose glands. The uterus has a very well developed muscular coat, a lymphoid mucosa without submucosa or muscularis mucosa, and long cylindrical glands. The mucosa of the Fallopian tube is thrown into branching folds, covered by cylindrical epithelium. The Fallopian tube opens into the peritoneal cavity at its outer end.

The lesions of the uterus are, the deformities already mentioned, inflammations, degenerations and tumor growths. We sometimes have inflammation limited to the mucous layer, endometritis; inflammation of the several layers, metritis; inflammation of the peritoneal covering, perimetritis; inflammation of the connective tissues adjoining the uterus other than the peritoneum, parametritis.

ACUTE METRITIS.

Synonyms: Puerperal fever; gangrenous endometritis.

Etiology: Some of the pus germs infecting

the uterus, either through tears in the cervix or elsewhere, or at the placental site.

Philosophy of the process: We can have infection through perineal tears; the route of infection here is through the inguinal lymphatics, for the vulva and the lower third of the vagina drain through the inguinal glands. Infection of the body through uterine tears spreads by the lymphatics, by the veins, and along the Fallopian tubes; the lymphatics of the vagina and the cervix drain to the hypogastric glands; the body of the uterus drains to the lumbar glands. Death may ensue from acute toxæmia without any lesion in other organs. We may have a slowly extending thrombus, giving phlegmasia alba dolens. We may have suppurative peritonitis, or pyæmia with multiple abscesses.

Anatomy: The uterus is enlarged, swollen, red, moist. The mucosa is thickened and injected. At the points infected there are large irregular ulcers, with ragged edges and yellow or black bottoms. Sometimes the veins leading from the uterus are thrombosed.

Histology: That of acute suppurative inflammation. The venous channels are filled with thrombi, and around these thrombi are the aggregations of round cells. The highly

specialized elements are in cloudy swelling and mucous degeneration.

CHRONIC ENDOMETRITIS.

Synonyms: Uterine catarrh; leucorrhœa; ulceration; erosion of the cervix; fungus endometritis; adenomatous endometritis; benign adenoma.

Etiology: There are two factors in the etiology of this affection, and the differences in these two factors are responsible for the wide variances in the disease. The first of these are infecting organisms; the second—changes in the host, by reason of which these infections become possible.

First factor: Gonococcus, streptococcus, staphylococcus, saprophytes, tubercle bacillus. These organisms either are in themselves milder than in the acute variety, or else there is a certain amount of acquired immunity.

Second factor: Subinvolution; ovarian disease; marked flexions; fœtal remains.

Philosophy of the process: It is never an endometritis, properly speaking, because there is no muscularis mucosa separating the mucosa from the uterine muscle. The veins, capillaries and lymphatics are continuous be-

tween the layers. The endometrium is simply
the seat of most marked inflammatory reaction. There is the usual piling up of lymph
tissue. The irritated glands may do one of
several things—some may undergo degeneration, and their epithelium becomes typical,
mucus secreting epithelium; some become
occluded and form cysts—such are the ovules
of Naboth; some of the irrigated glands make
new granular tissue. This process is the same
as the formation of new tubes in cirrhosis of
the liver, in ordinary adenoma, or in the adenoma due to coccidia; to this class belong
endometritis fungosa, hyperplastic endometritis, adenomatous endometritis. Coincident
with this development of tissue, there is necessarily a development of thin capillary vessels. There is the usual tendency of chronically inflamed mucous membrane, kept moist
to form polypi.

Anatomy: The uterus is enlarged, red, generally moist, and soft. Patches of red extend
from the cervix over the vaginal aspect. From
the cervix pours glairy muco-pus. On cut
surface the mucous membrane is greatly and
irregularly thickened and injected. The
mouths of the glands can be seen. In the
mucosa, and in the deeper structures, some

of these glands show as cysts as large as a pea, filled with thick mucus.

Histology: The apparent ulcers on the surface are wavy papillæ of spindle cells, covered by a single layer of columnar epithelial cells. The mucosa consists of round cells, imbedded in which are glands—some dilated, some normal in size. In older cases, between the gland tubes there are bands of old connective tissue. The findings vary so much in different sets of cases that an accurate description cannot be made to fit any number of consecutive cases.

TUBERCULOSIS.

The usual route of infection is via the vagina. It may come from fistula in ano, tubercular in origin.

Anatomy: The tubercles are found more frequently in the body of the uterus than in the cervix. The tubercles are along lymph channels in the deeper layers of the mucosa and in the muscular walls, the latter being the more frequent site. They ulcerate and discharge on the surface, giving irregular tubercular ulcers. They spread easily to the Fallopian tubes, ovaries, bladder, peritoneum, and later may become general.

SUBINVOLUTION.

Incomplete degeneration of the added elements of the uterus, after pregnancy and menstruation. It is accompanied by a growth of connective tissue and a chronic venous congestion.

TUMORS.

Polypus: A growth consisting of mucosa, uterine glands and blood vessels and covered by cylindrical epithelium. It springs from the mucosa exclusively. It is usually water soaked. It is usually pedunculated. It may be smooth or eroded or villous. It generally springs from near the cervix.

FIBROMYOMA.

Three varieties—according to location:

(1) Submucous, usually single, nonpedunculated, covered by areas of chronic endometritis.

(2) Intramural, imbedded in the uterine wall.

(3) Subperitoneal, usually multiple, globular, pedunculated. They sometimes become separated from the uterus.

These tumors grow to enormous size, or are present in large number.

Histology: There are bands of nonstriated muscle, and fibrous tissue, running in every

direction. They contain vessels with thick, rigid walls.

Degenerations: They are prone to cystic degeneration, when they may be converted into a single irregular large cyst; to calcareous degeneration; to infection, giving suppuration and sloughing; to ulceration, giving abundant hæmorrhage.

CARCINOMA.

May be of two varieties: (1) Carcinoma of the body, belonging to the class of cylindrical celled carcinomas. It rapidly passes to the Fallopian tube, or lumbar glands, or becomes general. (2) Of the cervix. This is squamous. The cervix may be hard and ulcerated, or it may be covered by fungous villosities. It is enlarged and hard and injected. The growth spreads to the vagina, the hypogastric glands, the uterine body, the neighboring organs.

SARCOMA.

Sarcoma of the vaginal portion gives a uterus that is enlarged and covered with a warty, villous growth. Microscopically, these villi are seen to be composed of spindle cells, covered by a single regular layer of epithelial

cells, columnar in type. In the body the sarcoma again has a tendency to a papillary surface structure. It is generally round celled in type. The cells grow from the mucosa and from fibrous tissue and from the muscle fibers of the uterine body.

A form of sarcoma, called deciduoma malignum, is found. In this the point of infection is the placental site. It occurs soon after labor when the uterus is still under the influences of the parturient state. There are present large decidual cells.

FALLOPIAN TUBES.

The arrangement of the epithelium of the tube gives a large amount of epithelial surface in a very small lumen. In consequence, there is frequent organic stricturing. Again, this long, delicate tube develops from one center, while its peritoneal covering develops from another. In consequence, the tube frequently kinks so as to form an occlusion of the tube. Again, this peritoneal covering is prone to adhesions, which furnish another source of stricturing.

SALPINGITIS.

Etiology: Streptococcus, gonococcus, staphylococcus, and other pus germs. These

germs spread from the uterus along the mucosa to the tubal mucosa (usual with gonococcus), or along the lymphatics from the lower regions. Stricturing with cystic accumulations forms a focus, inviting infection; abortion and miscarriage are the most frequent causes of infection.

Anatomy: There is considerable variation in the appearance of the tube, dependent upon the differing conditions bringing them about. It is tortuous; sometimes widely dilated, pear shaped and bound by surrounding adhesions. On cutting, sometimes clear water is found, sometimes pus, sometimes bloody water; sometimes the lumen is obliterated by a thick fibrous stricture; sometimes on straightening the tube, pus or serum can be squeezed into the uterus. The fimbriated end is almost always occluded. The wall is sometimes greatly thickened. This is due to an enormous overgrowth of circularly arranged, dense connective tissue. Sometimes the tubes are two inches in diameter. The thickening of fibrous tissue may be nodular.

Pyosalpinx is where the tubes are dilated by pus.

Hydrosalpinx is where the tubes are filled with albuminous water, derived either from the epithelium, or degenerated blood.

Infection of the peritoneum from suppurating tubes is habitual, until inflammation closes the fimbriated extremity.

Tuberculosis is frequent in the tube. It is found usually at the outer end as rather diffused tuberculosis of the submucous and muscular coats and neighboring broad ligament. It quickly infects the uterus, ovaries, and peritoneum.

The hydatid of Morgagni is a small retention cyst, hanging by a pedicle to the fimbriated extremity of the tube.

OVARIES.

Abscess of the ovary.

Acute inflammation of the ovary, other than suppurative in character, is seldom seen. The route of infection is along the tubes, either by the lymph channels, or by the mucous surface.

CIRRHOSIS OF THE OVARY.

Synonyms: Chronic interstitial oöphoritis; cystic ovary.

Anatomy: The surface of the ovary is very irregular. It is sometimes somewhat enlarged, sometimes it is small and corrugated. Multiple small cysts project from the surface.

It "cuts" tough. There are variously arranged bands of fibrous tissue, running in every direction. These enclose ovarian stroma, and in this stroma are cysts filled with clear fluid. These cysts are dilated or dropsical Graafian follicles.

Histology: There is little to be seen, save dense bands of fibrous tissue. Some of the follicles are cystic, while others are compressed and undergoing pressure atrophy.

TUMORS.

Cysts: The simplest cyst of the ovary is the dropsy of the follicles already mentioned. These are small and multiple.

OVARIAN CYSTS.

These are secretion cysts. The secretion is into the lumen of a previously formed adenoma. The cysts are always multiple to begin with. As they grow usually one cyst overshadows the others, so that we have an unilocular cyst. They attain very large size. The fluid may be mucus, serum, blood, etc.

Histology: Wall; young cyst, there is a fibrous tissue coat lined by columnar epithelium. Wall; old cyst, there is a fibrous tissue wall, in places thin, in places thickened. There is a varying amount of deposit of

fibrin on the inner surface of the wall. The epithelium is irregular in shape or amount or absent entirely.

PAPILLARY CYST ADENOMA.

A secretion cyst, developing in a previously developed adenoma. In this type there is a villous growth from the wall into the cyst cavity. After this arborization, covered by epithelium, has filled the cavity, it pushes its way through the wall opposite to that from which it springs, and appears on the surface of the ovary as irregular warts. These are easily detached. On whatever structure they fall they are prone to locate, and grow, giving villous tumors. They spring usually, though not always, from the hilum of the ovary, the epoöphoron, and grow into the ovarian structure.

Secondarily—These tumors cover the peritoneum, omentum, liver.

The ovary is a favorite site of dermoids.

Fibroma, myoma, chondroma, carcinoma and sarcoma are found in the ovary.

CYSTS OF THE BROAD LIGAMENT.

(Refer to embryology notes.)

Synonym: Parovarian cysts.

Philosophy of the process: There may be a retention cyst in Gärtner's duct. This may show in the walls of the vagina or uterus. The usual broad ligament cyst is in one of Rosenmueller's tubes. These run from the hilum of the ovary to Gärtner's duct. These cysts may be multiple or single, and occasionally are of large size. They have no pedicle. They are filled with a clear fluid. There are a few small tubes tributary to Gärtner's ducts that do not run toward the ovarian hilum. These are Kobelt's tubes. They are the seat of small retention cysts, with long pedicles.

THE NERVOUS SYSTEM.

POINTS IN HISTOLOGY.

The unit of the nervous system is the neuron. A neuron is a nerve cell with all its prolongations, both its axis cylinder and its shorter protoplasmic prolongations. The nerve fiber does not run direct into a second nerve cell, but encloses it in a basketwork of fine filaments.

The dura is a dense connective tissue layer. While it encloses large vessels it contains few vessels and few lymphatics. The pia is rich in blood vessels and in lymph spaces. Its vessels, lymphatics and connective tissue filaments run into the substance of the nervous tissues.

The vessels supplying the cortex are small in size and anastomose freely. The basal vessels are larger and do not have arterial anastomosis beyond the circle of Willis. It is well to bear in mind also that the basal areas belong to two classes, first, commissual, second, ganglionic presiding over coördination and the vital **processes.**

The meninges are subject to acute and chronic inflammation and tumor growths.

By reason of the different blood and lymph connections we have inflammations of the dura without pial involvement and vice versa.

Acute pachymeningitis.

Etiology: Sepsis, originating from injury to the scalp or skull, disease of the middle ear, infection from the venous sinuses.

Philosophy: There is more or less lymph connection with the cranial bones and through them into the neighboring cavities. It is possible to have an infection of the outer side of the dura without extension to its inner surface.

Anatomy: That of acute suppurative inflammation in the pleura, pericardium, etc., except that extravasation of blood is more prominent.

Pachymeningitis interna hæmorrhagica is a chronic inflammation with an abundant formation of granulation tissue. It corresponds to chronic pleurisy.

Leptomeningitis: Inflammation of the pia and arachnoid.

Varieties: Epidemic cerebro-spinal meningitis; suppurative meningitis.

Suppurative leptomeningitis.

Philosophy: The acute inflammations of the pia are productive, exudative in type, and are usually suppurative. There is a lack of relation between the post-mortem findings and the symptoms that is more marked in meningitis than in any other affection. This for two reasons: Firstly, the classical symptoms of meningitis are the results of cerebritis. Secondly, the toxins are found fresh and concentrated in the areas presiding over vital phenomena.

Etiology: Suppuration. 1. Neighboring, the middle ear, orbit, nose, scalp. 2. Distant, e. g., empyema. In the epidemic variety the pneumococcus has been found most frequently.

Anatomy: The effusion is more frequent at the base, where it tends to accumulate under the cerebellum around the pons in front to the longitudinal sinus and laterally into the Sylvian fissures. The ventricles may be filled. The effusion into the ventricles frequently exists without involvement of the base and vice versa. There is the same lack of connection with the convexity. The remaining anatomy and the histology are the same as in typical suppurative inflammation in serous **structures.**

Tubercular meningitis.

Philosophy: This is a disease of childhood. It is nearly always located in the pia. It is a blood vessel infection. It is found nearly always at the base. Along the Sylvian artery and its branches, the surface of pons and bottom of the cerebellum are the areas of selection. Dural tuberculosis and occasionally pial tuberculosis may arise from bacilli in the skin, nose or eye, being transported by lymphatics.

Anatomy: The distribution of the nodules along the arterioles and venules of the base has already been outlined. There is extensive effusion into the great lymph space of the base and into the ventricles. This is largely a passive transudation due to obliterating lesions in vessels. This is sometimes so considerable as to be termed acute hydrocephalus. The possibility of secondary infection and its changes are to be remembered.

Histology: The lesions are generally of the round cell type. Reticular tissue and giant cell formation is exceptional. The small nodules of endothelial cells may be due to proliferation of the cells of the intima, of the adventitia or of all the coats.

Syphilis.

Philosophy: It is usually a dural disease. It is most frequently in the shape of a solitary gumma. From pressure the cranial bones become porous and disappear in the areas of pressure. If the syphilitic lesion begins on the inner surface of the dura, it projects into the brain area, flattening the substance. A gumma primary in the brain substance is rare.

The histology of gumma has already been studied.

Hydrocephalus: May be congenital or acquired.

Congenital hydrocephalus.

Anatomy: The ventricles are widely dilated and filled with clear fluid. The brain substance is thin, compressed and with only rudimentary convolutions. The cranial bones of the vertex are thin. The sutures and fontanelles are so wide that the cranium bulges, giving the appearance of overhanging the face and neck.

THE CEREBRUM.

It is well to study the cerebrum as composed of parenchyma (the brain cells and those portions of the cells called fibers) and interstitial tissue.

The Parenchyma: Our known technical methods are of very little service in showing affections of the cells of the nervous system. We know of fatty degeneration, and vacuolation of the nucleus. We are not able to satisfactorily distinguish cloudy swelling or the phenomena of productive inflammation in the parenchyma. That they exist is beyond doubt. A perverted chemistry in a nerve cell will give expression to a symptom far more promptly than in any other structures.

ACUTE DIFFUSE INFLAMMATORY PHE-
NOMENA.

Histology: The nerve cells are rounded in shape. Their nuclei may be vacuolated; there is a diminution in the number of protoplasmic processes which can be demonstrated; the fibrous prolongations are swollen, making globular colloid looking bodies. The neuroglia and pial connective tissues are proliferating.

Abscess of the brain.

Two Varieties.

1. Pyæmic abscess.

Etiology: Infection with some of the pus germs through the circulation.

Anatomy: These abscesses are multiple,

of small size, and death ensues before there is evidence of more than slight pus formation.

Second Variety: In this the infection is from without through lymph connections or lymph connections in greatest part.

Etiology: The most frequent cause is suppuration of the middle ear; then in about the following order, trauma, suppuration in the nose, orbit, scalp—unknown.

Anatomy: Generally speaking, there is a single large abscess with green or gray pus and a ragged soft wall in the vicinity of the point of infection. In cases of trauma without fracture, and in some cases of otitis media the abscess is some distance away from the surface and the point of infection and no route of infection can be demonstrated.

INTERSTITIAL TISSUE.

The interstitial tissue is of two types. The neuroglia tissue derived from the epiblast, the ordinary connective tissue derived through the pia from the mesoblast. This includes the vascular and lymph vessel supply.

Scleroses.

Varieties: Diffuse; multiple.

Diffuse. In old people there is an overgrowth of connective tissue that is diffused

throughout. The convolutions are flattened; the membranes are thickened. The attachment of the dura to the calvarium is more close than normal. There are isolated cases in people other than the aged.

Multiple Sclerosis:

Philosophy: The process is the same as sclerosis in other organs. What determines the location other than its arrangement with regard to blood vessels is as unknown here as elsewhere. It is subject to the same serous infiltration and to colloid or mucoid degeneration.

Anatomy: Irregularly placed in the brain and cord are irregularly shaped patches that are gray in color. They are sometimes hard and sometimes soft, waxy and translucent. They blend insensibly into the surrounding tissue. They are not raised above the surface, but rather depressed.

Histology: That of cirrhosis. Bands of fibrous tissue enclosing atrophying, degenerating nerve elements.

Disease of the vessels.

Apoplexy: Hæmorrhage into the brain as a result of rupture of a vessel.

Etiology: There is always disease of the arteries; atheroma or miliary aneurism.

Philosophy: The effects are divided into

primary and secondary. Both depend in great measure upon the areas into which the effusion takes place. The secondary effects depend upon the fact that the nerve fiber is a part of the nerve cell, and any part of a cell separated from its nucleus dies. If the cell is in the cortex the areas of secondary death are below the injury. If the cells are in the medulla or pons, etc., the areas of secondary death are above. These are called respectively descending degeneration and ascending degeneration.

The first effect is an outpouring of blood proceeding until clotting stops the vessel, or until external pressure equals internal. The area of hæmorrhage breaks down into granular debris. At the periphery, where there is blood supply intact, there is reactive inflammation. This may build up a cyst wall and liquefaction proceeding in the center a cyst may result. The surrounding fibrous tissue and vessels may grow into the clot organizing it and giving an area of sclerosis. The waters of the area may absorb and leave a caseated mass behind.

Descending degeneration: When the nerve fiber is separated from its nucleus it dies throughout its length. To illustrate: A

hæmorrhage into the internal capsule would give degeneration of the crusta of the crura, anterior pyramids of the pons and the medulla, the direct and crossed pyramidal tracts in the cord, to the anterior horns. Here they form a plexus around the motor cells and end. Therefore degeneration ends.

The histological phenomena are: Formation of colloid masses in the axis cylinder processes, globular aggregations of fats in the white substance of Schwann, overgrowth of connective tissue, converting the area into a fibrous patch.

Thrombus: A clot *in situ.* This forms more frequently in the carotid artery.

Embolus.

Etiology: A clot or vegetation from some larger vessel. It may be composed of fat in lipæmia, or of other foreign matter. It may be infected.

Philosophy: The vessel generally occluded is the middle cerebral, because it gives a nearly straight course from the heart. As this vessel is a terminal artery, the area supplied by it undergoes starvation necrosis. Whether the area is to be pale or red depends upon principles already discussed. Its anatomy, histology and secondary degenerations are similar to those of apoplexy.

THE SPINAL CORD.

The inflammations of the chord are acute and chronic.

The acute inflammations termed myelitis are somewhat better known than those of the brain, because the cord is much more accurately mapped out.

Myelitis shows the same phenomena already described in cerebritis. There is congestion of the vessels, both of the pia and of the cord substance. The cells are rounded, granular, poleless. There is breaking down of the protoplasmic processes. There is production of round cells by the connective tissue and exudation from the vessels. In transverse myelitis the process affects a transverse section of the cord. There is secondary ascending and descending degeneration in the cord.

Anterior poliomyelitis: Synonyms. Infantile paralysis. Acute atrophic paralysis.

Etiology: Intoxication, sometimes from absorption from the intestinal tract, sometimes of unrecognized origin. Exposure to cold. This last probably acts by locating an irritant already absorbed or causing the absorption of an irritant already produced.

Philosophy: The process nearly always

begins as an acute infection accompanied by
the phenomena of acute toxæmia. During
this stage the lesions are those of myelitis,
limited to the anterior horns. With the subsidence of the intoxication the disease is,
properly speaking, at an end. Such of the
cells as are not irretrievably injured return to
the normal. Those that are injured beyond
repair are absorbed by the leucocytes. The
protoplasmic processes of those cells degener-
ate. There is an overgrowth of connective
tissue. The degeneration involves the anterior
roots of the nerves and the nerves themselves.
The muscle fibers supplied by the cord at
that level atrophy, not only from disuse, but
also from having their trophic center destroyed, it being in the anterior horn of gray
matter. The muscles are the seat of fibrous
tissue overgrowth.

Anatomy: A cord, years after primary
lesion. The gray matter of the affected half
of the cord, when it is a hemiplegic lesion, is
markedly decreased in size. This gray matter is translucent. The changes are not in
continuous areas, but in disconnected foci.
The half of the cord is decreased markedly in
size.

Histology: In acute stage the histology is

that of acute myelitis limited to the anterior horns and to the protoplasmic prolongations of their nerves. In the wake of the disease we find connective tissue overgrowth and atrophy of the parenchyma elements, both from pressure and from inflammation.

Chronic interstitial myelitis: According to the location in the chord of this cirrhosis we may have multiple sclerosis, antero-lateral sclerosis, amyotrophic lateral sclerosis, or locomotor ataxia, glosso-labial paralysis.

We will study locomotor ataxia.

LOCOMOTOR ATAXIA.

Synonyms: Tabes dorsalis, posterior spinal sclerosis.

Etiology: Obscure; syphilis, lead poisoning, sexual excess.

Philosophy of the process: The cells of the posterior columns are located either peripherally or on the ganglia of the posterior roots. Perhaps there is sometimes primary disease in these ganglion cells, and perhaps the disease is an inflammation of the meninges at the point of entrance of the posterior roots, but at any rate the lesions of tabes are those of degeneration in nerve fibers separated from their nuclei. The degeneration enters the cord

by the posterior root zone, travels from there to Goll and Burdach, thence across the posterior horn, where some of them surround cells and end; others run to the direct cerebellar tract, the ascending, lateral and mixed lateral columns and anterior horns.

Anatomy: The meninges are thickened and adherent, especially in its posterior segment. The posterior portions of the cord, especially in the lumbar region, are flattened. Cross sections show the posterior columns, the seat of grayish, gelatinous looking, fibrous tissue. Less well marked areas are seen in the lateral columns. The extent of the lesion becomes less as we proceed toward the medulla.

Histology: That of degeneration of parenchyma and overgrowth of connective tissue.

Tumors of the brain and cord.

Fibroma, endothelioma, glioma, sarcoma, carcinoma, cysticercus, echinococcus, cholesteatoma. Some claim all gliomata to be sarcomata.

In spina bifida there is an imperfect closure of the vertebral bones posteriorly and generally at the base of the cord. Through the opening the cord prolapses. It may hang intact, but usually there is varying degree of deformity.

DISEASES OF THE BLOOD.

Points in Histology: The blood is a meso-blastic tissue. It differs from other tissues in that there is more intercellular substance than usual, and this intercellular substance contains more than the usual quantity of water. The cells are the red cell, the white cell and the third corpuscle. The red cell is a non-nucleated mass of protoplasm containing hæmoglobin. Its sole capacity is that of a gas transporter. The white cell contains no hæmoglobin. In the mature state it has a nucleus surrounded by granular protoplasm. Each cubic millimeter of blood contains 5,000,000 red cells and 5,000 to 10,000 leucocytes and enough plasma to make up the volume.

The organs to be studied in connection with the blood are the spleen, the bone marrow, the lymph tubes, and probably also the endothelium of the vessel.

The spleen: The spleen consists of a connective tissue framework and of spleen cells. These spleen cells are in two groups. First,

Malpighian corpuscles. Second, the spleen pulp. The smaller arteries are surrounded by Malpighian corpuscles, then the blood flows among the spleen cells, then being gathered up into venous radicles, then veins. In the spleen pulp the blood is free among the spleen cells. The area between the arterial and the venous radicle is a pulp space.

ACUTE SPLENIC TUMOR.

Synonyms: Active hyperæmia of the spleen; acute splenitis.

Etiology: All toxæmias, e. g., malaria, typhoid, typhus, scarlet fever, smallpox, pyæmia and septicæmia.

Philosophy of the process: The spleen being both a chemical filter and a source of leucocytes, it rapidly responds to the irritation of the poisons on which it acts, for the fact that it acts on those poisons is proof that it is susceptible to them.

Anatomy: The spleen increases to as much as four times the normal size. The capsule is tense. The substance is soft, diffluent, chocolate brown in color, and rapidly oxidizes to a brighter red. It may seem creamy, almost pus-like.

CHRONIC INTERSTITIAL SPLENITIS.

Etiology: Malaria; rickets; syphilis.

Philosophy of the process: That of cirrhotic lesions elsewhere. The spleen is the chief source of destruction of the malarial organism. This is accomplished by the endothelial cells of the trabeculæ and lymph spaces. This mild irritation, when continued, results in cirrhosis; at the same time there is accumulation of pigment granules, derived from the blood.

Anatomy: The spleen is enlarged, firm. The capsule thick. It cuts firm. The color is pale except in the malarial, when there is pigmentation.

Histology: The trabeculæ are increased in thickness. The blood vessels have thickened walls. The pulp spaces are decreased in size and the connective tissue wall is thickened. In this wall contained within cells are granules of golden brown pigment.

WAXY SPLEEN.

Synonym: Sago spleen.

Etiology: Same as waxy disease elsewhere.

Philosophy: As the spleen is a blood structure it is a very frequent seat of waxy infiltration. The deposit may be principally

in the corpuscle, in which event the sago appearance is most marked, or else it may be in the walls of the pulp spaces, when the appearance is somewhat different.

Anatomy: The spleen is enlarged, firm, elastic, with rounded edges. On section the corpuscles look like grains of boiled sago. The spleen pulp is pale, gelatinous. Iodine stains the amyloid brown; the other areas yellow.

Histology: The waxy homogeneous areas map out the trabeculæ and the blood vessel wall. The staining reactions are the same as waxy degeneration elsewhere.

THE PLASMA.

The plasma is at once the source of nutrition and the sewer channel for the body. Therefore it will not be inappropriate to describe the post-mortem findings in certain diseases that are purely toxæmias, in which the organism may be in the plasma, in which, certainly, the toxin is in the plasma, and in which death ensues without production of special lesion in any organ. To this class would belong septicæmia, typhus, yellow fever, cholera.

Post-mortem findings: Cadaveric rigidity

is early and well marked. Putrefaction begins early. The blood is dark and fluid.
There is much evidence of staining of the
vessels and surrounding tissue with blood.
The lungs are congested. The same is true
of the meninges. There may be fluid in the
ventricles. There are usually small petechiæ in the gastro-intestinal and bronchial
mucosæ and in the serous membranes, the
meninges, pericardium, pleura, etc. There
is swelling of the glands of the ileum and of
the mesenteric glands.

Scurvy: Purpura hæmorrhagica; hæmophilia.

Scurvy is a nutritional disease in which
some of the organic salts of the plasma are
deficient. It seems probable that potassium
enters into this combination. It is characterized by a diminution of the tendency to coagulation, but less marked than in the next two
members of the group.

Purpura hæmorrhagica: This condition is
merely symptomatic. It is found in many of
the prolonged toxæmias. There is a diminished tendency to coagulation.

Hæmophilia: This disease may be congenital or acquired. Its subjects are recognized as "bleeders." The blood has lost all

tendency to coagulate. The plasma is entirely free from calcium salts. The assimilation of calcium is curative. With the return of calcium to the plasma the capacity to coagulate is regained.

Diabetes: In diabetes mellitus the percentage of sugar in the plasma rises from one-tenth of one per cent to six-tenths of one per cent. This causes an absorption of water from the tissues and the blood becomes hydræmic. In turn the kidneys secrete an excess of urine and the specific gravity of plasma arises. In diabetes sometimes the amount of suspended fat so increases as to give the condition known as lipæmia.

THE RED CELL.

Each cubic millimeter contains 5,000,000 red cells. This we term 100 per cent. A certain shade of color, as determined by a scale of comparison, we term 100 per cent of hæmoglobin. Now, then, if 100 per cent of red cells carry 100 per cent hæmoglobin, each corpuscle carries its normal load or 100 per cent. This is called the corpuscle index.

The red blood cell in adult life is manufactured in the bone marrow almost exclusively. An ordinary nucleated connective tis-

sue cell containing no hæmoglobin divides and produces a new cell, which has the capacity of taking up hæmoglobin. This cell is large and nucleated. This divides and forms a small cell seven mikrons in diameter, containing a nucleus and charged with hæmoglobin. This in turn loses its nucleus and assumes the shape of the red cell. It is the red cell. Normally no red cells appear in the blood stream except the completed product. In times of emergency all or any of these elements may be rushed into the blood current.

Anæmias divide themselves along lines of etiology into those that are hæmogenic, and those that are hæmolytic. To the former type belongs chlorosis. To the latter pernicious anæmia.

	Number of red cells per ctm.	Percentage.	Percentage of hæmoglobin.	Corpuscle index.
Immediately after 10 per cent hæmorrhage	5,000,000	100	100	100
One day after 10 per cent hæmorrhage	4,000,000	90	90	100
Chlorosis	4,000,000	80	40	50
Pernicious anæmia	1,250,000	25	30	120
Normal blood	5,000,000	100	100	100

The above is an illustrative table. The loss from hæmorrhage is purposely made large. These figures in chlorosis and pernicious anæmia are very frequently found.

Anæmia after hæmorrhage: As plasma, red and white cells are lost in the same proportion, each cubic millimeter of blood contains the same relative amount of plasma. red cells and hæmoglobin and leucocytes as in health. Immediately fluids begin to soak in from the tissues. In consequence each cubic millimeter contains a large quantity of plasma and a small quantity of red cells and white cells. The white cells are formed with great rapidity, so that within a few hours there is a post-hæmorrhagic leucocytosis. The low specific gravity and the changed chemistry of the plasma causes a destruction of some of the red cells and a loss of hæmoglobin that is still more marked. Next the marrow supplies new red cells, generally non-nucleated, but some nucleated, and all deficient in hæmoglobin. So that the percentage of hæmoglobin falls below the percentage of red cells. We have a low corpuscle index. This is not to be confounded with chlorosis. Later the hæmoglobin rises to the normal. The small nucleated cell present is called a

normoblast. The large nucleated cell, rarely present, is called a gigantoblast or megaloblast. The bone marrow normally yellow becomes red.

Chlorosis: If the percentage of red cells stays above 80 the disease is termed chlorosis. If it falls below 80 it is termed chloroanæmia.

Etiology: Absorption of ptomaines from the gastro-intestinal tract. It is especially a disease of constipated women, breathing bad air and removed from the effects of sunlight.

Philosophy: It is a hæmogenic disease. The urine is pale, indicating that the amount of coloring matter manufactured from the blood is not in excess of the normal.

Examination of the blood: The blood count shows a high corpuscle percentage, a low hæmoglobin percentage, a low corpuscle index. Examination shows pale corpuscles, irregular in size and in elasticity; a very few normoblasts. The specific gravity is low; 1,035-38 is about an average. Leucocytosis is absent.

PERNICIOUS ANÆMIA.

This is only a symptomatic disease. The primary disease is chemical and is located

somewhere in the portal circuit, the area of both normal and pathological hæmolyses.

Etiology: Ptomaines absorbed from the gastro-intestinal tract. Whether there is a special germ manufacturing a special ptomaine, or whether there is change in the alimentary tube by which an ordinary germ is provided with a medium from which it can manufacture a special ptomaine, or whether the absorptive apparatus is so changed that it takes up a ptomaine usually rejected, or whether the liver fails to destroy a ptomaine that is normally destroyed, we do not know.

Philosophy of the process: It is a hæmolytic disease. The urine is highly colored, indicating that there is increased destruction of hæmoglobin. We are to bear in mind that 20 per cent hæmoglobin should mean one-fifth the normal coloring matter in the urine. The urine contains an increase of aromatic sulphates and is rich in pathological urobilin. The blood gives every evidence that hæmogenesis is making a gigantic effort to compensate.

Blood Examination: The blood shows a small percentage of red cells, a small percentage of hæmoglobin, a high corpuscle index. Note this. The index ranges very close to

100, and it may go considerably over it. The red cells are variable in size, shape and elasticity. Large cells called macrocytes predominate. Normoblasts and megaloblasts are both present. No leucocytosis. In extreme cases there may be an apparent, though there is no real leucocytosis. Fibrin formation takes places more rapidly than normal.

The White Cell: The white cell is certainly manufactured by the lymph tubes and glands and probably also by the spleen, and, possibly, by the endothelium of the vessels. It is a mesoblastic cell that wanders in and out of the blood current with so much of facility and is so closely related to other mesoblastic cells that likewise wander, that it is easy of study, but difficult for satisfactory conclusions. It begins by fission of mesoblastic cells outside the blood current. In the blood current it does not divide. The new cell is small, about 8 μ, consisting of a central nucleus and a very faint small rim of non-granular protoplasm surrounding. This acquires protoplasm, making a larger cell about 10 μ in size. This protoplasm becomes filled with fine granules that stain with neutral stains, and at the same time the nucleus twists into

an irregularity of design, giving the idea of multiple nuclei. These so-called polynuclear neutrophiles make up 60 per cent of the whole number. The small lymphocyte makes up 30 per cent, and the other 10 per cent is furnished by the intermediate stage by eosinophiles and basophiles. The eosinophile is a large cell with a simpler or twisted nucleus and filled with large granules resembling vesicles that stain with an acid stain, e. g., eosin. Rarely we find a cell with granules staining with a basic stain such as methylin blue. These are basophiles and are closely akin at least to the "mast" cells of the tissues, and especially of the gastro-intestinal tract. The fact that the number of corpuscles can multiply several fold in a few hours would indicate that any percentage here is rather haphazard.

In addition to the above there is a cell of great diagnostic, though not pathognomonic, significance. It is called the myelocyte. It is the largest of all the cells, averaging 15.7 μ. The large twisted nucleus neutrophiles average 13.5 μ. The myelocyte has a single large oval nucleus, generally eccentrically placed. The nucleus stains evenly. The cell protoplasm is granular. The granules are, gener-

ally speaking, fine. They are neutrophiles, that is, the granules stain with a combination of an acid and a basic stain.

Leucocytosis: A temporary increase in the number of leucocytes. It is purely symptomatic. The term can be applied to either an increase in the whole number of leucocytes, or to an increase of some special variety or stage.

Physiological leucocytoses:

1. Leucocytosis of the newborn.
2. Leucocytosis of digestion.
3. Leucocytosis of pregnancy.
4. Leucocytosis of puerperal state.
5. Leucocytosis after violent exercise, massage and cold baths.
6. Leucocytosis of the moribund state.

Pathological leucocytoses:

1. Post-hæmorrhagic leucocytosis.
2. Inflammatory leucocytosis.
3. Toxic leucocytosis.
4. Leucocytosis in malignant disease.
5. Other leucocytoses.

Post-hæmorrhagic leucocytosis. Within an hour after hæmorrhage the number of leucocytes may rise to 18,000 per cm. This, though the hæmorrhage be inconsiderable.

Inflammatory leucocytoses:

1. Infection mild; resistance good; small leucocytosis.

2. Infection less mild; resistance less good; moderate leucocytosis.

3. Infection severe; resistance good; marked leucocytosis.

4. Infection severe; resistance poor; no leucocytosis.

Infectious disease giving leucocytosis: Asiatic cholera, relapsing fever, typhus, scarlet fever, diphtheria, follicular tonsilitis, syphilis (secondary stage), erysipelas, bubonic plague, pneumonia, smallpox, pyæmia and septicæmia, actinomycosis, trichinosis, glanders, acute multiple neuritis, beri beri, acute articular rheumatism, cerebro-spinal meningitis empyema of the gall bladder, acute pancreatitis, endometritis, cystitis, gonorrhœa, abscesses of all kinds, including appendicitis, pyonephrosis, osteomyelitis, psoas and hip abscess, salpingitis. Inflammations of the serous membranes, gangrenous inflammations. Many inflammatory dermatites, pemphigus, herpes zoster, prurigo, and some cases of universal eczema.

Toxic Leucocytosis.

Causes: Illuminating gas, quinine, rickets, gout, acute yellow atrophy, advanced

cirrhosis, acute gastro-enteritis, acute nephritis, hydronephrosis, tubercular and thyroid extract injections, after injection of normal salt solution, salicylates, ether.

Diseases in which there is absence of leucocytosis: Typhoid fever, malaria, grippe, measles, rötheln, all forms of tuberculosis.

LEUKÆMIA.

Etiology: Not known.

Varieties: Lymphatic; spleno-myelogenic.

1. Lymphatic leukæmia.

Blood: The percentage of red cells is about 50, and that of hæmoglobin somewhat lower. There are nucleated reds, both normoblasts and megaloblasts present, though they are not prominent.

White cells: The average number of whites is about 150,000 per cm.; about 90 per cent of the white cells are small lymphocytes under 10 m. in size. Myelocytes are rare. Plasma coagulation delayed.

Body: The lymph glands are diffusely enlarged. The enlargement is due to true lymph gland overgrowth. There is but slight enlargement in the spleen.

2. Spleno-myclogenic leukæmia.

Blood: Red cells. The red cells average

about 60 per cent, and the contained hæmo-globin somewhat less. These will depend very much upon the amount of hæmorrhage. Hæmorrhage is prominent in this affection. There is a great increase in nucleated reds, especially the normoblast.

White cells: The number of white cells is increased to from 100,000 to 1,000,000 per cm. The increase is principally in the so-called polynuclear form and in the myelocyte. These average as high as 30 per cent of all the forms. The small lymphocyte is relatively diminished.

The plasma is very slow to coagulate.

Body: The spleen is enormously over-grown. While there is a moderate increase in the connective tissue, the main increase is in the lymph elements, especially those filling the pulp spaces. The bone marrow is red. Petechiæ and punctate hæmorrhages are fre-quent.

The parasites of the blood are:

1. Animal: Malaria (the red cell); filaria sanguinis hominis; distoma hæmatobium.

2. Vegetable: Spirochæte of Obermeyer; anthrax; pus germs, etc.

POINTS IN ANATOMY AND HISTOLOGY OF THE TEETH.

The roots of the teeth are in sockets in the alveolar processes. These alveolar processes are merely ridges on the maxillary bones. Binding the teeth to the bone is a peridental membrane composed of white fibrous connective tissue, many lymphatic glands and many blood vessels. The tooth proper is composed of an enamel which is epiblastic in origin, a dentine which is mesoblastic in origin, a cementum which is due to ossification of those portions of the peridental membrane next the dentine. Therefore the centers of development of a tooth are enamel, epiblast, dentine, mesoblast, cementum mesoblast through peridental membrane. Centers of ossification of the alveolar processes of the maxillary bones. Upper incisor for the four incisor teeth; palatal for the remainder of the teeth. This would mean four centers in all. Lower, one for each side, two in all. The pulp is made up of connective tissue,

blood vessels and nerves. Both of these
leave the bone at the apex of the socket,
give off lateral branches to the peridental
membrane, then enter the tooth at the apex
of the root. Neither runs into the dentinal
tubules.

FORMATION AND ERUPTION OF TEETH.

Calcification of the deciduous teeth begins
with the crown of the central incisors during
the seventeenth week of fœtal life, and ends
with the second molar and canine of twenty-
two months after birth. During this time
any severe constitutional strain will show itself in abnormalities in these teeth. Calcification of the permanent teeth begins during
the twenty-fifth week of fœtal life and ends
at the twelfth year of post-fœtal life. These
teeth are subject to the same laws of nutrition
as their predecessors.

Eruption of the deciduous teeth is hastened
by nutritional diseases and especially by
rickets.

Eruption is delayed by grave systemic disease or by a lack of vitality. As a general
proposition delayed dentition is not as sig-
nificant as premature dentition.

TARTAR.

By this is meant the deposits on the teeth above the gingival border.

It is composed of the solid ingredients of the saliva combined with food remnants and a rich growth of bacteria. It accumulates on the teeth because they are subject to less irrigation and friction than the balance of the mouth. It is, generally speaking, most abundant on those teeth placed near the outlets of salivary ducts—e. g., the second molars of the upper jaw; the central incisors of the lower jaw.

Fresh tartar is soft, moist, yellowish white, and offensive in odor.

Microscopically: It is composed of granular debris, epithelial cells and bacteria of various kinds.

Old tartar: Is firmly adherent to the enamel; so much so that considerable force is necessary to remove it. It is black or dark brown in color. It may extend below the line of gum attachment. This is not the rule.

Microscopically: It is composed of lime salts and bacteria. Tartar is only of importance in that it is generally though to predispose to decay. When the accumulation of

tartar becomes large the condition is known as salivary calculi. Cases are not exceedingly rare in which masses fill the roof of the mouth, completely hiding the teeth. The masses are bone-like in appearance. Chemically they are composed of sodium carbonate potassium sulpho-cyanide, calcium salts, ptyalin and occasionally uric acid.

DECAY.

Synonym: Caries.

There are many points in dental caries that are not yet solved, and that will not be solved soon. Many of these questions hinge on (1) why infection takes place, and (2) the relation of germs to germs. Both questions are difficult of solution. As the enamel is by all conceded to be relatively passive, by nearly all to be absolutely passive, the question resolves itself into three suppositions. First, that the proper germs do not happen in the mouth until a certain time. This is improbable. Second, that certain resident germs that combat the germs of decay fail to do their work. Third, that there is some change in the chemistry of the secretions of (1) the mouth, (2) the enamel plate, or (3) the intercellular substance, so that they fur-

nish a feeding-place for the germs of decay. This is probable.

Etiology: Two sets of causes.

1. Immediate. Two varieties of germs are needed, one living largely on starches and sugars secretes lactic acid, which dissolves the lime salts in all the structures of the tooth; a second living on albuminous foods, and following in the territory previously prepared by the first. It secretes a ferment which digests the epithelium of the enamel plates and the connective tissue of the dentine and cementum.

2. Remote. Illy formed teeth. Illustrations. Fissures and depressions in teeth so placed as to be protected from friction; badly placed teeth by making cleansing difficult; recession of the gums. Diseases—rheumatism, gout, diabetes, dyspepsia, cancer of the stomach, rickets, scrofula, tuberculosis, syphilis. Occupations—bakers, confectioners. The carbohydrates furnish food for the growth of the lactic acid germ.

Location: The most frequent point of beginning is in a fissure or depression on the grinding surface. Next in frequency comes the spaces between the teeth, then the labial, lastly the lingual surface. Caries beginning

in the cementum covering the root is rare, even in cases of marked recession.

Nature of the process: The area to be affected is covered by a layer of germs secreting acids. These decalcify the enamel, and the germs grow into the enamel area as slender rows parallel with the long diameter of the enamel plates. These rows extend until the dentine is reached, when the germs get into the dentinal tubules. In these tubes they grow with greater rapidity. Following close behind this advanced guard is an organism or a set of organisms secreting a substance which digests the organic parts of the structure. In the dentine both of these processes extend more rapidly than in the enamel. In consequence the enamel is undermined, and crumbles off. In the cavity thus formed many kinds of germs multiply. Some are chromogenic, giving the black color; some secrete odoriferous gases, giving the odors of decomposition; some are actively pyogenic. When these last secure entrance to the pulp chamber or to the peridental membrane, there is pus formation; abscess. Sometimes the pyogenic germs are either gas producers, or are associated with saprophytic germs producing gases: the ab-

scess contains both pus and gas. Infection may extend to the bone, causing necrosis that may be extensive.

Anatomy: In the very beginning the enamel has lost its polish; it is whiter than its surrounding. It is slightly roughened. Later a cavity is formed. This cavity is globular in shape, being larger below than on the surface. The wall is rough. It is some dark shade of color.

Histology: Enamel. Rows of some form of bacillus or coccus are seen extending between the enamel plates. The plates are granular, disintegrating and falling loose from their fellows and from the basement membrane underneath.

Dentine: Masses of organisms are seen especially in the dentinal tubules, and less frequently in the interglobular spaces. The areas deprived of lime salts show anatomically as softened gelatinous areas. Histologically there is slight change in appearance. Later the dentinal structure begins to break down into granular debris, some of it passing through the stages of cloudy swelling and fatty degeneration. In the vicinity of the breaking down process the dentinal tubules are filled with proliferated osteoblasts or with secondary dentine produced thereby.

Pulp: When the germs reach the pulp cavity we may have chronic pulpititis with formation of secondary denture and lessening of the cavity, or suppuration, or suppuration with formation of gases, all of these being dependent upon the infecting germ.

EROSION.

This is a condition in which on surfaces not exposed to wear depressions, generally angular and clear cut, appear. The term is not applied to the wear resulting from use.

Etiology: Unknown. It is found in people subjected to severe, long continued illness or great mental strain. It is not a common effect of these conditions, but is seldom found unassociated with them.

Anatomy: On the labial surface, most frequently in the enamel, but sometimes on the root there appears a depression giving every appearance of an area of wear. The loss is usually about one-third the diameter of the tooth. The bottom is smooth, polished, firm.

Histology: Except for a thickening of the dentine and a lessening of the pulp chamber, I have been unable to find any changes in the few cases that I have examined.

TEETH OF SYPHILIS.

Hutchinson's teeth. In the permanent teeth of the subjects of inherited syphilis the grinding surfaces have a large single crescentic notch.

Teeth of rickets: In either set of teeth, but especially in the milk teeth, there are changes due to rickets. The teeth are yellow, soft and porous. They begin to decay very early and decay with great rapidity.

Any severe disease causing profound disorder of nutrition affects the teeth as to their time of eruption, their placing, the development of the dentine and of the enamel. The teeth are most subject to these changes during their formative period. The milk teeth would be most affected by intrauterine conditions and affections during the first year. The permanent teeth by affections during the first and second and up to the tenth year of life.

Diseases of the pulp cavity: The pulp chamber is, properly speaking, nothing more than that portion of the tooth organ which has not been converted into dentine by the odontoblasts. Any irritation that is mild is liable to cause proliferation of odontoblasts and the formation of new dentine. This may

proceed until the pulp chamber is obliterated, either at some point or throughout. As a matter of fact, the size of the pulp chamber varies greatly at different periods of life. Such a production of dentine can clearly be classed as a chronic productive inflammation of the pulp; a chronic interstitial pulpitis. In the same area are large cells called odontoblasts that cause absorption of dentine and a consequent increase in the size of the pulp cavity.

Infection of the pulp chamber: Route of infection. Through decay in the enamel and dentine.

Etiology: Some of the pyogenic germs frequently associated with gas producers.

Nature of the process: Pulp cavity is intensely inflamed. The inflammation extends to the apical foramen. The pus germs may cause liquefaction of the peridental membrane, when the pus will appear at the side of the tooth, or it may remain at the apex liquefying the bone. Infection of the lymph spaces of the bone may ensue, causing necrosis of considerable areas. General infection may result. The production of gases is the rule.

Histology: The pulp is filled with round cells of inflammation. Among these are large

giant cells called odontoclasts that are lique-fying the dentine. Around the apex and the lymph spaces leading therefrom are masses of inflammatory cells.

Sequelæ: An apical abscess may terminate by phagocytes overcoming the infecting germs. It may infect the peridental membrane, giving pyorrhœa alveolaris, beginning at the apex of the root.

Sometimes tumors are found in the pulp. These may be fibromata, or they may be deposits of lime salts—odontoliths.

Diseases of the peridental membrane: The blood and lymph supply of the peridental membrane is from two principal sources. First, branches of the vessels to the tooth at the apex; second, branches from the gingival border.

PYORRHŒA ALVEOLARIS.

Synonym: Rigg's disease.

Definition: A chronic inflammatory process located in the peridental membrane, resulting in disintegration of those fibers running into the cementum.

Etiology: Anything causing mild, chronic irritation, such as deposit of inorganic salts, continued irritation of the gums, lead and mer-

cury poisoning, scurvy. If this area becomes infected with pus germs either down the gingival border, or at the apex through the pulp, the process is greatly hastened. Decay plays very small part in the process.

Anatomy: The teeth are usually sound. The loosening usually takes place from the neck toward the apex. This shows as a roughened area. This area may be broad, or it may be in striæ running lengthwise of the root. There are generally deposits of mineral matter in this area. Beyond the zone of loosening there may be deposits, but this is exceptional.

Histology: The peridental membrane is filled with round cells. In some cases this round cell infiltration and proliferation are evenly distributed throughout. In other cases it is collected in multiple foci. In many of these foci there is granular degeneration of the inflammatory cells (atheroma) with secondary deposit of lime salts (calcification). The process is very similar to that in periostitis and in arteritis. In this connection study those conditions carefully. To this class belong "serumal calculi." Beyond a slight amount of mechanical injury the calculi do no harm.

MERCURY POISONING.

In poisoning by mercury there is an acute inflammation of the peridental membrane followed generally by pus infection.

Etiology: Certainly some part of the mercury in the system is eliminated by the salivary glands and other structures of the mouth. This fact means special irritability. The infection follows because the inflamed area is one of lowered resistance.

Anatomy: The gums are swollen, soft, red œdematous. The tooth is partially loosened. Frequently pus exudes.

Histology: The peridental membrane is the seat of acute productive exudative inflammation. Its meshes are filled with round cells. Sometimes foci of pus are to be seen.

LEAD POISONING.

Poisoning with lead gives about the same anatomical and histological findings. Generally speaking, the process is less virulent and less acute than that of mercury.

In scurvy much the same findings are seen.

DISEASES OF THE GUMS.

The gums consist of stratified squamous epithelium arranged over papillæ. They

cover the peridental membrane. Around the neck of the tooth the cells take on a somewhat glandular arrangement. These cells resemble those of sebaceous glands. It is this collection of cells called the glands of Serres that is most sensitive to mercury, potassium iodide, lead and scurvy, and therefore they are the starting point of the disease in the underlying structure. The gums cannot be treated apart from the peridental membrane, because the capillaries, blood vessels and nerves are continuous between the two. The gums are the more subject to pathological processes, because

1. Epithelium is the more irritable tissue.

2. Its position subjects it to mechanical, chemical and bacterial irritations. From the gums start the larger number of cases of pyorrhœa alveolaris.

THE MOUTH.

The more important inflammations of the mouth are aphthous stomatitis, thrush, ulcerative stomatitis, gangrenous stomatitis, diphtheria, follicular tonsillitis, syphilis.

Aphthous stomatitis: Etiology not known. Several germs have been cultivated from these "ulcers," but the probability is that the main cause lies in some change in the general economy through which these cells become subject to infection with germs omnipresent.

Philosophy of the process: A mild inflammation causing destruction of superficial cells, proliferation of deeper cells, but limited to the epithelial structures and the connective tissue immediately underneath.

Anatomy: Generally the ulcers are pea size, white, rough, with a red setting.

Histology: Proliferation of granular layer of epithelial cells, with mild infiltration of underlying connective tissue with inflammatory cells.

Thrush: A form of superficial stomatitis affecting bottle-fed babies especially.

Etiology: Oïdium albicans, a mold feeding especially on sugars and starches and mycoderma vini, a yeast.

Philosophy of the process: A mild irritant causing inflammation limited to the epithelial structures. If the irritation be more severe, it may involve the mucosa underneath the epithelium.

Anatomy: The mucous membrane is injected. On this red base is a white membrane which scrapes off easily, leaving a slightly roughened surface.

Histology: Among the loosened and the proliferating epithelial cells are cells and branching threads of the yeast or mold.

ULCERATIVE STOMATITIS.

Synonym: Cancrum oris.

Etiology: Pus infection, due to poor hygienic surroundings.

Anatomy: The lesion begins in the gums. From around the teeth pus oozes; the teeth are loose; parts of the bone may necrose and come away. The mucous membrane of the gums and cheeks sloughs away. An exudate of plasma and leucocytes mixed with tissue debris partly covers the raw surface.

Histology: That of suppurative inflammation in mucous membranes.

In gangrene of the mouth, called noma, the process is the same, except that the infecting germ is one of those causing gangrene.

DIPHTHERIA.

Synonym: Membranous croup.

Etiology: The diphtheria bacillus.

Philosophy of the process: This bacillus, more than any other, causes exudation of plasma. It is then violently irritative to the vaso-motor apparatus. In addition, it has capacity to coagulate albumins in a much more marked degree than have the toxins of most germs.

The lesions of diphtheria are of three classes.

1. Local: An exudative inflammation with coagulation not only of the exudate, but also of every tissue cell in close proximity to the toxin.

2. General: Due to the absorbed toxin.

3. Secondary infections—e. g., pneumonia.

Point of infection: Area of selection, the tonsils. It may begin in, or it may spread to the nose, the pharynx, larynx, trachea, œsophagus, eyes, skin, rectum, vagina, anus.

Anatomy: The mucous membrane is red and swollen. The diphtheritic membrane is

white to gray in color. It is closely adherent. A bleeding surface is left when it is removed. It is usually on the tonsil, but it grows out over the surrounding mucosa.

Histology: The superficial layers consist of fibrin, coagulated cells and bacilli. The deeper layers show cells separated by bands of coagulated fibrin. Deeper there is violent round cell inflammation.

Constitutional lesions: As a rule, the bacillus does not go beyond the area of infection. Its toxin absorbs, causing cloudy swelling of the kidney, cloudy swelling of the liver, cloudy swelling of the heart, neuritis.

Complicating lesions: The paralyses are due to the toxæmia. The diphtheritic throat is a good growing area for other germs, and these inspired are apt to cause either broncho or lobar pneumonia.

FOLLICULAR TONSILLITIS.

Ulcerations of the throat.

Etiology: The pus cocci.

Philosophy: In the crypts of the tonsils one or more of these germs grow in rich profusion, secreting toxine, which is absorbed, causing the symptoms.

Anatomy: The white masses, generally

speaking, grow as islands and are limited to the tonsil. They are easily scraped off. The mucous membrane is red and swollen.

SYPHILIS.

We may have a primary chancre, a mucous patch or a gumma. Syphilitic teeth have already been referred to. The lesion of syphilis is an overgrowth of fibrous tissue in the submucosa. There may or may not be necrosis, ulceration.

As we consider the lesions of the mouth, remember that the mucous membrane of the mouth is continuous with that of the nose, pharynx, larynx, œsophagus, Eustachian tube and ear, eye, frontal sinus and antrum of Highmore. Into this last occasionally the roots of the first and second molars penetrate.

The bones: The alveolar portion of the superior maxillary bone developing from two centers for each half, and the inferior maxillary from one for each side, the upper teeth are more subject to irregularity than are the lower.

Abnormal forms of arch. U-shaped, in which the arch is too broad. V-shaped, in which the two sides form a V with the angle in the center. Saddle-shaped arch, in which

there is an angle pointing inward just external to the lateral incisors. Irregular placing or spacing is found in all of these.

Frequently the alveolar process is not long enough to hold all the teeth, when crowding and irregularity ensue.

TUMORS OF THE MOUTH, JAWS AND TEETH.

Cysts: Retention cysts are not unusual in the glands accessory to the mouth. Dermoid cysts are not infrequent in the face and mouth. Sites—angles of the orbit, upper eyelid, along the nose, chin, angle of the mouth, tongue. Branchial cysts, due to imperfect closure of the branchial clefts. Sites —the ear, and in the neck along the anterior border of the sterno-mastoid muscle.

Epithelioma: The carcinomas of the mouth are epitheliomata. In the tongue they are virulent; in the lips they are but mildly malignant; in the gums they occupy middle ground.

Epulis: Most of the tumors of the maxillary bones that were formerly called epulis belong to two classes:

1. Giant celled sarcoma. This springs from the peridental membrane or the alveolar process. It has been described under tumors.

2. Cysts developing as a perversion in a tooth organ. These develop around perma-

nent teeth. Less frequently from undeveloped teeth.

Anatomy: There is a thin envelope of osteosclerotic bone around the cyst. This is globular in shape. Within this is a thin connective tissue wall, and within this clear fluid. In the cyst is found some part of a tooth.

Bone is subject to (1) necrosis or simultaneous death of a considerable mass of bone.

(2) Caries: Ulceration of bone. Solution of lime salts liquefaction of the connective tissue framework. The irritant of the latter is the more violent.

Osteosclerosis is that condition in which osteoblasts form a greater quantity of bone than normal or fill up the Haversian spaces more completely than normal.

Osteoporosis is that condition in which the phagocytic cells called osteoclasts have absorbed some bone either in the central canal at the periphery, or in the Haversian spaces.

Generally speaking, when in an area of concentrated irritation osteoclasts are causing absorption in surrounding areas of lesser irritation; osteoblasts are laying down new dense bone.

www.ingramcontent.com/pod-product-compliance
Lightning Source LLC
Chambersburg PA
CBHW020902210326
41598CB00018B/1746